PENGUIN BOOKS
FITNESS SECRETS OF THE STARS

Born in Kolkata, Ram Kamal Mukherjee started his career as a film journalist twenty years ago with the *Asian Age*. Later, he shifted base to Mumbai and worked with publications such as *Stardust*, *Mumbai Mirror* (the Times of India Group), *Mid-Day*, *Anandabazar Patrika* and the TV18 group. He headed *Stardust*—India's leading film magazine—as its editor-in-chief. He also has a popular Sunday column—'Ram Katha'—in *Mumbai Mirror*, and has hosted the Bengali chat show *Talk Bangla*, which featured thirteen Bollywood celebrities. In 2005, Ram authored a coffee-table book on Hema Malini, *Diva Unveiled*. He was the vice president of Pritish Nandy Communications for over a dozen feature films. He co-produced the Hindi TV show *Bin Kuch Kahe* for Zee TV in 2016, and published his first work of fiction, *Long Island Iced Tea*, in the same year. His authorized biography of Bollywood's legendary actress Hema Malini, *Beyond the Dream Girl*, has fetched him national and international accolades.

Devyani G. Ghosh's interest in writing goes way back to her schooldays in Baghdad International School, Iraq, where she won a prize in a prestigious international essay contest in the tenth grade. The scholarship money from the contest funded her English (honours) education in Presidency College, Kolkata. During her last year in college she interned at the *Asian Age* and discovered that journalism was her calling. Working at the *Indian Express* in Mumbai and, later, being the Mumbai correspondent for the *Pioneer*, Delhi, brought her into close contact with the world of Bollywood, as did a short stint as an interviewer with Zee Music.

FITNESS SECRETS OF THE STARS

RAM KAMAL MUKHERJEE
AND
DEVYANI G. GHOSH

BLUE
SALT

PENGUIN BOOKS

An imprint of Penguin Random House

PENGUIN BOOKS

USA | Canada | UK | Ireland | Australia
New Zealand | India | South Africa | China | Singapore

Penguin Books is part of the Penguin Random House group of companies
whose addresses can be found at global.penguinrandomhouse.com

Published by Penguin Random House India Pvt. Ltd
4th Floor, Capital Tower 1, MG Road,
Gurugram 122 002, Haryana, India

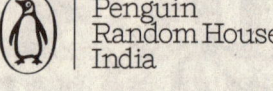

First published in Penguin Books by Blue Salt Media and
Penguin Random House India 2018

10 9 8 7 6 5 4 3 2

While every effort has been made to verify the authenticity of the information
contained in this book, the publisher and the authors are in no way liable for the
use of the information contained in this book.

ISBN 9780143425854

Typeset in Sabon by Manipal Digital Systems, Manipal
Printed at Repro India Limited

www.penguin.co.in

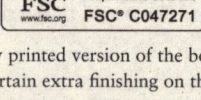

To Nari Hira, my mentor, and chairman
and founder of Magna Publishing. This book
wouldn't have been possible without you.

To all aspiring actors and models
who dream of becoming a star.

And to Hussain Zaidi who has been instrumental in
making this project possible.

Contents

Acknowledgements   ix

Introduction   xi

1. Hrithik Roshan: A Lean, Mean
   Fighting Machine   1

2. Challenging All Fitness Limits:
   The Aamir Khan Way   27

3. Priyanka Chopra: Bold and Beautiful   51

4. Varun: Dhawan and Only   69

5. Farhan Akhtar: Body and Brains   91

6. Tiger Shroff: The Sculpted Dancer   115

7. Bipasha Basu: Abs-olutely Gorgeous   135

8. Shahid Kapoor: Fiery and Fit   157

9. John Abraham: Body of Work   183

10. Sonu Sood: The Indian Arnold
    Schwarzenegger   203
11. Dev: God from the East   225

Notes   241

Acknowledgements

Ram

I would like to thank the well-known veteran author and my ex-colleague Mr Hussain Zaidi for believing in us. He has set a benchmark when it comes to patience, and definitely deserves an award for his perseverance.

We are eternally thankful to all the trainers of the superstars featured in the book for helping us out with the right information about the stars (who are generally quite secretive). Though some of them made us chase them, some were cooperative, while others ducked our questions. But these are the challenges one usually faces while dealing with the crème de la crème of Bollywood.

This book wouldn't have been possible without the cooperation of media mogul Mr Nari Hira from

Magna Publishing. Mr Hira allowed us to access the archives of *Stardust* and *Health & Nutrition* magazines for the finer details on many actors featured in this book. He also gave us permission to use images from the *Stardust* archives for the book.

I would also like to extend my grateful thanks to my wife, Sarbani Mukherjee, and friend Saheli Mitra for burning the midnight oil with me in research and editing.

Devyani

This book was a pleasure to write as I was privy to so much valuable information. I would like to thank Hussain for considering me for this book and thus providing me with the opportunity to become an author—something I've wanted to be for a long time.

I would like to thank Ram for being my co-author in this creative and purposeful journey.

I would also like to thank my dear son, Aniruddha, for helping me out with the technical difficulties relating to my iPad, which facilitated the writing process!

Introduction

Today, fitness has become an intrinsic part of our daily lifestyle. Joining a gym, taking a Zumba or yoga class or even marathons on a regular basis is the norm in many urban cities. In Bollywood, too, it has become a necessity. Through our experiences—one of us is the editor of India's leading film magazine, *Stardust*, while the other is a former senior journalist at the *Indian Express*—we have seen actors slowly and steadily understand the importance of having a fitness plan, hiring trainers and adopting diets for different roles.

There was a phase when actors like Hrithik Roshan, John Abraham and Salman Khan were known for flexing muscles and flaunting their muscular torsos, but there were also actors like Shah Rukh Khan, Akshay Kumar, Saif Ali Khan and Ajay Devgn who didn't believe in showing off their bare bodies. They were fit, but not necessarily muscular. By the early 2000s, fitness was no longer an option, as it had been till then. The media played a vital role in highlighting the workout regimens of actors, and most magazines featured their bodies prominently. Soon, everyone wanted well-defined muscles and six- or eight-pack abs. From Shahid Kapoor to Varun Dhawan, from Vidyut Jammwal to Tiger Shroff, everyone developed enviable physiques.

This book is the brainchild of the author and our friend S. Hussain Zaidi. He wanted us to write a book that focused on the workout and diet regimens of Bollywood celebrities. As both of us had closely followed the fitness trends that had taken over not only Bollywood but also the youth of the country, we decided to delve deeper into the subject. And thus we set off on a rollercoaster ride to track down the trainers of these superstars from the local movie industry.

While working on this book, we realized that all the featured actors have maintained an extremely disciplined life to achieve what they did. But almost all of them have trusted fully in their trainers, who have been elevated to the status of sculptors capable of creating magic with their tools. If Hrithik Roshan looks like a Greek god on-screen, a significant amount of credit goes to Satya, his trainer, for sculpting his body so.

Though all actors take this part of their job very seriously, at the same time they use it to balance their love for food. Most actors are big foodies. We know for a fact that Salman Khan loves biryani, while Hrithik goes weak in the knees when it comes to chocolate. Dev, aka Deepak Adhikari, Bengal's undisputed superstar, loves to eat Kolkata-style mutton biryani. Again, Bipasha is a hardcore foodie and her weakness is chocolate. But all of them know how to burn the extra calories they consume in the gym. So, those who think actors don't eat or that they live off protein powders and shakes are far from the truth. We hope this book serves as an eye-opener for those who have been following a restrictive diet in the pursuit of achieving a body like their favourite superstar.

We realized there are many aspiring actors across the country who believe that achieving a good body is easy and is the only prerequisite for being a successful actor. I have interacted with people who could barely speak a grammatically correct sentence in Hindi or English but wanted to be actors because they had good bodies. Even if you consider just looks, having a good body is not enough. Looking good on-screen requires one to have a *great* body. People don't know the amount of hard work these actors put in just to achieve those well-defined muscles.

Writing this book also reinforced the idea that all stars are under constant peer pressure. If a certain actor is seen doing a romantic scene in a swimming pool, then his or her contemporary would also want to flaunt his torso or her lean physique in a similar scene.

Through this book, we have strived to provide detailed information about the diets and fitness routines of film's brightest stars. We reveal to you the little tricks and tips they have to keep their weight down and morale high. For example, Farhan Akhtar is a sports addict. Shahid Kapoor is a diehard vegetarian and feasts like a king. But at the end of it, they are all extremely motivated, disciplined and focused individuals. Priyanka Chopra is holistic in her approach, so she is more partial to yoga rather than a hardcore gym workout.

This book is meant to reach out to people who want to follow the same workout routines as their favourite stars as well as those who want to make their fortunes in showbiz. There are many who stay in the dingy lanes of Mumbai's suburbs, work out at local gyms and give auditions at Adarsh Nagar in the hope of pursing their dreams as aspiring actors. But as is evident from all the unique and varied training details outlined in the book, body sculpting is an art.

Everybody is different, and so is every trainer. Though this book fleshes out almost all the secrets of a superstar's regimen, we earnestly request and recommend everyone to consult a physician and personal trainer before aping any actor's workout and adhere strictly to what Varun Dhawan said during one of his shoots for a *Stardust* cover: 'Steroids are a complete no-no, it might give you a quick result but the after-effect is life-threatening.'

The book includes not just the workouts of Aamir Khan, Hrithik Roshan and John Abraham but also of young heart-throbs like Varun Dhawan and Tiger Shroff. To make the scope wider, we also have inputs about Dev, who underwent rigorous training for his blockbuster *Chaamp*. Bipasha Basu, along with Esha Deol and Shilpa Shetty, started the trend of washboard abs for female actors. They set the trend for an entire generation of female stars, who are still following in their footsteps.

So grab your gym gear and settle in for an adrenalin-filled journey!

1

Hrithik Roshan: A Lean, Mean Fighting Machine

Bollywood Background

Bollywood has been lucky to have its very own mortal Greek god in Hrithik Roshan since 2000—chiselled features, a sculpted physique, effortless grace, high-voltage energy and dreamy blue-green eyes to boot.

But apart from his stunning features and body, it is his superlative acting talent that makes Hrithik a natural superstar. Who can forget his first impactful performance in *Kaho Naa . . . Pyaar Hai* (2000), his debut film, for which he received several awards? Rohit and Raj, the two characters he played with such charm and intensity, instantly made him the heart-throb of the nation. This combined with his mind-blowing moves during the dance sequences catapulted him instantly into the category of iconic dancers in Bollywood.

In 2001, he appeared in the family drama *Kabhi Khushi Kabhi Gham*, which became India's highest-grossing film in the overseas market.

He also gave some noteworthy performances in the commercially successful *Koi Mil Gaya* (2003) and its sequel Krrish series, which won him numerous best actor awards.

Hrithik received his third Filmfare Award for best actor in 2006 for his performance in the action film *Dhoom 2*.

In *Krrish 3*, the actor stunned the audience with some superb stunts and superhero moves. His adrenaline-pumping action moves created celluloid magic for a wide-eyed kiddie audience, who found in Krrish a local superhero they could compare to Superman. A lot of little boys all over the country were demanding to be fitted into flying capes and black masks after watching the movie. His stunts, combined with a super-toned body, created a powerful impact.

Hrithik's stunning physique was the result of his incredible commitment and dedication to a high performance workout routine that has stood him in good stead over the years.

Hrithik's Fitness Mantra

Hrithik is very committed and dedicated to his fitness regimen. His fitness mantra is based on two words: initiative and consistency.

His trainer, Satyajit Chaurasia, or Satya, as everyone calls him, admires Hrithik's unwavering focus and discipline. He's been with him since 2004 when Hrithik shot for *Lakshya*.

Satya maintains that working out is like an addiction for the actor. As a popular health icon and actor with a large fan following, the pressure to look good at all times is tremendous. Although at times he slacks a bit on his diet and does not work out every day. While on vacation or travelling, Hrithik might go two to three weeks without working out. But that said, three to four months before a film shoot he's at his most serious and dedicated best with regard to working out.

But in spite of that, Hrithik is able to achieve an incredible physique in a very short time, for every movie. The reason behind this, says Satya, is that 'Hrithik's body has very good muscle memory. His body is magical. It takes him only a month or so to get back in perfect shape'. Within one to two months of intense training he's able to work off all the body fat and hone it into lean muscle.

Muscle memory is a very important factor in strength training and a durable fitness routine. It is the long-term effect of previous training on muscle fibres that the muscles 'remember'. This is true of many athletes who undergo strength training, and experience a rapid return of muscle mass and strength even after long periods of inactivity.

Hrithik has a well-defined workout routine to increase stamina, endurance, flexibility and give his body that athletic look combined with a muscular physique. The tough workout and fitness regimen that he has been following consistently over the years has ensured that he has one of the best bodies in Bollywood. His discipline is to be admired as his is ability to bounce back in spite of tremendous adversities.

Overcoming Adversities

'I have become a star not in spite of my weaknesses, but due to them,' says Hrithik. It takes hard work, dedication and unflinching determination to achieve perfection. Lumps of coal become diamonds. Grapes become expensive vintage wines. Iron becomes steel. So it is with Hrithik. From being a traumatized child with a speaking disability to becoming a superstar with millions of fans, Hrithik has come a long way.

Speaking about his childhood, he says he was bullied by his peers for having a stutter. His inability to speak properly gave him nightmares. 'For oral tests at schools, I used to bunk school, I used to fall sick, I used to break my hand, I used to get a sprain.' One can only imagine the kind of trauma a young boy must have faced in such situations. And this same boy has now attained superhero status.

Doctors and speech therapists helped, but only to an extent. What helped him most was his own unstinting effort and determination to overcome his disabilities.

When he was twenty-one years old, he was diagnosed with scoliosis, a sideways curvature of the spine that occurs during the growing years just before puberty. While scoliosis can be caused by conditions such as cerebral palsy and muscular dystrophy, the cause of most scoliosis is unknown.

He was told by one of the best doctors in the country to not take up acting as a profession, as it would put a lot of physical strain on his spine and this could put him in a wheelchair for life. He remembers it as a 'big blow' but he then continued to work positively to make his dream of becoming an actor come true.

Misfortune struck again in 2010 when he was diagnosed with a bad knee, due to years of wear and tear on account of dance practice for five to seven hours daily. The condition had apparently made his left knee more brittle than an old man's. Despite his grim condition that worried his doctors, the actor did not give up.

In July 2013 the *Krrish* star was diagnosed and treated for a brain clot. But Hrithik again acted like a superhero and tweeted before going in for surgery: 'Minor brain surgery to remove blood clot. Should be rock n rolling by evening. U guys have a great day too! Supersonic!! [sic].'

His father, Rakesh Roshan, also an actor and well-known director of the Krrish series and *Koi Mil Gaya*, commented, 'He hit his head during the shooting of *Bang Bang* in Phuket. The doctors believe the reason for it was that he had been shooting many action sequences. Around two months ago, he leaped from a height of 30 feet and sustained an injury while falling on a water body.' This diagnosis was given by the actor's consultant neurosurgeon. But some months after his surgery, the actor developed excruciating back pain. This was so severe that he was unable to sit in the same position or even the same seat for more than thirty minutes. Around 2013–14 he faced another major setback in his personal life: legal separation from his wife, Sussanne Khan, and the mother of his two sons, Hrehaan and Hridhaan.

He probably learnt how to deal with such adversities since childhood. In 2000, a life-changing moment had occurred for Hrithik when his father was shot. He felt completely powerless when he saw him in the hospital. It forced him to introspect. From that point, he adapted to the idea that although some situations can be disheartening, they also provide an opportunity to learn and grow. It's what led him to always put in that extra effort and keep going even in difficult times.

The positivity that this brave heart actor sends out is tremendous. His ability to bounce back from misfortunes time and again is phenomenal. Hrithik's take on life is very simple but profound: 'When it comes to fitness, I'll propagate just two magic words, which have helped me tremendously. First is "initiative". You need to take that first step . . . The second magic word is "consistency". Even if you are taking baby steps, take it every day. Do something for five minutes, but do it every day.'[1]

Body Issues

Hrithik has had to struggle a lot to build muscle because he has an ectomorph body type, which does not put on weight easily and has a very high metabolism. It has taken years of dedicated training to build up muscle mass. Also, Hrithik's long history of injuries meant that a lot of care had to be taken regarding the type of exercises that he could or couldn't do,' confides Satya.

He also admits that apart from taking years to build the kind of body Hrithik has, it's also a struggle to maintain it, as it requires a lot of consistency and effort.

The Basic Diet Plan that Hrithik Banks on for a Fab Body

Satya confides that Hrithik loves to eat and try out new food. Satya remembers the time they were in the US for two months, Hrithik frequented a lot of restaurants and enjoyed a variety of cuisines like Italian, Mexican and Japanese. He loves Japanese food, which is quite healthy and tasty. Hrithik's all-time favourite is biryani, which according to Satya he can indulge in quite frequently, and he thoroughly enjoys desserts too. But he still prefers healthy alternatives. He loves chocolate, which he gorges on, especially as a midnight snack! But he makes sure he sticks to a proper diet plan when the time comes for him to do so. So although he is a foodie and gives in to his cravings, he's always very regular with his workouts that help keep him in shape. Satya says of Hrithik's eating habits: 'After all, eating also releases endorphins or feel-good hormones in the body, so why should Hrithik be expected to follow a strict diet every day?'

Moreover, Hrithik knows all the tricks to balance out any excess fat or grease-laden food that he might have consumed during the day. He either cuts down portions later in the day or next day. Or he has cups of black coffee, green tea or hot water to tackle the fat in his body. Then, he burns fat in a cardio workout the next day.

Satya's advice is not to cut down on eating. Enjoy your food but balance it out by exercising regularly. Maintain a proper workout schedule and if you play sports then do so on a regular basis as this will also release endorphins in the brain which make you feel good. To acquire a body like Hrithik's, follow a regular workout plan and maintain a healthy diet. 'Slow and steady wins the race' is his essential advice. Consistency is important, he adds.

About three to four months before a shoot, Hrithik follows the proper diet plan that Satya has prepared for him. This gives him the energy required to sustain his intense workouts and also maintain the muscle mass that he builds.

He has five to six meals in a day at specific times depending on his body requirements, energy expended, and so on, and consumes about eight to twelve egg whites in a day across these meals. This along with some fish or chicken meets his protein requirements for the day. Satya explains that protein intake for a person is measured according to their body weight. So, ideally one should have proteins according to this calculation: 1 kg = 2.2 pounds. When you multiply your weight with 2.2, the resulting amount in grams should be your daily protein intake. Hrithik weighs 75 kg, so he has 75 x 2.2 = 165 g every day. Or, depending on his weight then, he uses this measuring method to ensure optimum protein intake.

The first thing that Hrithik consumes in the morning is a bowl of citrus and other fruits, which gives him his required dose of vitamin C. He has a litre of water along with this. After working out for an hour in the morning, he has a protein shake. For breakfast, he has about four to six egg whites that are prepared as a 'bhurji' with veggies, and two slices of multigrain bread. Satya stresses that it is very important to eat carbs during the day to keep energy levels high. You cannot cut off carbs completely from your diet, else you will not be able to go about your daily activities. At night you can have a low-carb meal or avoid carbs altogether. During shoots, Hrithik follows this rule very strictly.

For lunch, he has about 70 g of chicken or fish along with a bowl of steamed white rice and lots of veggies and salad. Although brown rice is healthier, the actor prefers white rice. While Hrithik has the option of eating rotis as well, he prefers rice. Given this option of choosing between rice and rotis, he's able to enjoy his meals more.

After his evening workout, which is for about two hours, Hrithik has another protein shake. His dinner is the same as lunch—but without any roti or rice. All portions throughout the day are strictly measured in grams.

Even if Hrithik does eat out during these three to four months before shooting, he requests the restaurant chef to prepare the meal according to his dietary requirements. All his meals are cooked in minimum oil and salt, and spices are avoided. Hrithik also totally cuts out sugar during this time.

He eats every three hours. This is essential to maintain muscle mass, says Satya. Another trick used by him is to consume a lot of protein in order to consolidate muscle mass, especially in the form of whey protein shakes. He increases his intake by a glass or two in the months before shooting begins. But one has to be very careful to not have too much protein if not expending a proportional amount of energy.

Also he prefers to eat more fish than chicken as fish meat is leaner and easier to digest. This contributes to developing a lean and sleek muscular body faster. He totally abstains from alcohol, avoids junk food and smokes only occasionally. He also increases his veggie intake which helps him to feel full faster due to its fibre content. This meal plan has stood him in good stead over the years.

His exercise routine is also more intense at this time. He trains twice a day. He does cardio for thirty minutes in the morning with abs. In the evening, he focuses on two body parts for one and a half to two hours.

From Fat to Fit

There was a phase in the actor's life when he sank into a hugely unhealthy lifestyle. 'I was doing too many things at a time—a TV show, a huge film. All that then ended up becoming toxic for my body. I had developed a double slip disc. It eventually progressed to bed rest for a couple of weeks. Then there was the

stress of shooting another film. I began smoking . . .
I put on a lot of weight. I was so unhealthy that I
couldn't even lift my son.'[2]

He needed a complete transformation as he was
also scheduled to shoot for the Krrish series. He had
a 36.5-inch waist. He could not get his superhero
jacket on. He was suffering from blood pressure
issues. He had been lying flat on his bed for months
and gorging on cupcakes, brownies and chocolates
brought by well-meaning family and friends. Add to
this feeding frenzy a smoking habit, which meant he
went through almost three packs a day for two and a
half years. All this took a major toll on his physique
and he needed a drastic change to come out of it. But
who would help him with this?

After months of concentrated research and
initiative, he found the answer in Kris Gethin, a
trainer from the UK. Hrithik took the similarity of
Kris's name to his character's in *Krrish 3* as a sign
and decided to work with him. Thus began his
journey to transform himself.

Hrithik's Magical Transformation

Surprisingly, Hrithik was able to spring back into
shape within the next ten weeks, even though Kris
had scheduled twelve weeks for the transformation.
After ten weeks of intensive training, Hrithik went

from a 36.5-inch waist to 30 inches, losing 10 kg in the process. One must not forget that Hrithik's body has incredible muscle memory.

His high metabolism, which his trainer boosted, helped him lose the weight faster. Hrithik says, 'I was force-fed till I was stuffed . . . My metabolism became high. Because my metabolism was high, I started losing weight. I was burning calories faster.' The more he ate of the right food, the more it boosted his metabolism.

Nutrition Plan

During this period, Hrithik changed his nutrition plan weekly, keeping his health condition and weight in mind. Kris also took heed of Hrithik's blood type and insulin sensitivity when he made his diet chart. But there were some recurring patterns in the plan. His staple foods for the day consisted of 100 g meat, fibrous carbs like broccoli, sprouts and spinach, and a cup of rice or pasta. But these foods were all steamed, boiled or sautéed.

His protein came from:
- Protein powder
- Steak
- Turkey
- Fish

- Egg whites

His carbs came from:
- Brown rice
- Oatmeal
- Pasta
- Salads

Hrithik's Supplement Support

Hrithik had pre- and post-workout shakes were mixed with a whey protein supplement and walnuts or oats in a smart shaker. He also had protein shakes either as a meal substitute or before bed.

Morning:
- L-glutamine
- BCAA (branch chain of amino acids)
- Anavite supplement
- Grapeseed antioxidant
- Omega-3
- Liver detoxifier

Before cardio:
- Pre-workout energy drink

Pre-Workout:
- Optimum-nutrition BCAA

- Nutrition anavite
- Thermo detonator
- Grapeseed antioxidant

Post-Workout:
- Whey protein supplement
- L-glutamine
- Optimum-nutrition BCAA

Before bed:
- ZMA
- Casein protein
- Glutamine/L-glutamine
- BCAA
- Omega-3
- Grapeseed antioxidant
- Liver detoxifier

Hrithik's Training Regimen

A lot of CrossFit sessions were incorporated into his workout as he had to be athletic and also prevent getting injured. He did twenty minutes of cardio after breakfast, which involved swimming, beach walking, running, CrossFit and various cardiovascular exercises. This was repeated after the evening workout as well.

His workout for the week looked like this:

Day 1: Chest, Back and Calves

- Dumb-bell bench presses
  - Warm-up sets of 6–10 reps
  - Working sets of 6–10 reps

- Incline dumb-bell presses
  - Sets of 8–10 reps

- Underhand cable pull-downs
  - Warm-up sets of 8–10 reps
  - Working sets of 8–10 reps

- Bent-over barbell rows
  - Warm-up sets of 8–10 reps
  - Working sets of 10–12 reps

- Hyperextensions (back extensions)
  - Warm-up sets of 10–12 reps
  - Working sets of 10–12 reps

- Seated calf-raises
  - Sets of 20 reps

- Standing calf-raises
  - 3 sets of 18–20 reps

Day 2: Legs

- Leg presses: 10–12 reps (4–5 warm-up sets); 10–12 reps (3 working sets)
- Seated leg-tucks: 15 reps (2 warm-up sets); 12–15 reps (3 working sets)
- Lying leg-curls: 15 reps (2 warm-up sets); 12–15 reps (3 working sets)
- Leg extensions: 15–20 reps (2 warm-up sets); 15–20 reps (3 working sets)
- Hack squats: 15–20 reps (2 warm-up sets); 20–30 reps (3 working sets)

Day 3: Rest

Day 4: Shoulders, Abs and Calves

- Seated barbell military-presses: 6–8 reps (2 warm-up sets); 6–8 reps (3 working sets)
- Side lateral-raises: 12–15 reps (1 warm-up set); 12–15 reps (3 working sets)
- Upright barbell rows: 7 reps (3 sets)
- Reverse flyes: 12–15 reps (7 sets)
- Weighted sit-ups with bands: 15–20 reps (3 sets)
- Seated calf-raises: 20 reps (3 sets)
- Standing calf-raises: 18–20 reps (3 sets)

Day 5: Arms

Straight-arm dumb-bell pull-over: 10–12 reps (2 sets)

- Cable rope overhead tricep extensions
  - 10–12 reps (3 sets)
- Cable lying tricep extensions
  - 10–12 reps (3 sets)
- Standing bent-over one-arm dumb-bell triceps extensions
  - 10–12 reps (3 sets)
- Straight-arm pull-downs
  - 10–15 reps (7 sets)
- Concentration curls
  - 12–15 reps (2 warm-up sets); 12–15 reps (3 working sets)
- Dumb-bell alternate bicep-curls
  - 12–15 reps (2 warm-up sets); 12–15 reps (3 working sets)
- Standing biceps cable curls
  - 15–20 reps (3 sets)

Hrithik's Health Tips

1. Almost 90 per cent of the job is done through your diet. The other 10 per cent is exercise. You are what you eat.
2. If you miss meals and stay hungry, you tend to opt for pizzas and/or burgers. This messes up the

body. So stay away from junk food and instead eat healthy meals.

3. Street food, packaged food, and ready-made meals are bad. Anything with preservatives is unhealthy. Try to eat fresh home-cooked meals.

4. Curb or completely do away with addictions like cigarettes. Nicotine is more addictive than cocaine. So stay away from these substances.

Vitamins and Supplements

1. Multivitamins with breakfast

2. He consumes 10 gm of BCAA in 1 litre of water while working out, to keep himself supplied with energy. But one can have this as a pre- or post-workout supplement. This is the perfect supplement for people looking to build up muscle mass. This supplement also boosts your energy levels.

3. 5 g L-glutamine are his after-workout supplements along with a whey protein shake. But Satya does not think it is advisable or needed to take these vitamins separately as most whey protein powders contain BCAA and glutamine. Also if one is not working out intensely, then extra supplements are not required. Also the vitamins and supplements that Hrithik used during his Kris Gethin transformation phase were quite hardcore, according to Satya, and do not need to be taken

on a regular basis. They are to be taken upon recommendation or for a short duration only.

Basic multivitamins and protein supplements are what Hrithik has throughout the year.

Hrithik's Regular Workout Routine

1. He begins with 5 minutes of stretching.
2. He moves on to 10–20 minutes of cardio, choosing from cycling, the treadmill or elliptical trainer.
3. Then workout for 1.5 hours.
4. And then 20 minutes of cardio.

Cool-down stretches for 5 minutes He focuses on two body parts every day for two hours:

- Monday: Arms (biceps and triceps)
- Tuesday: Chest and back
- Wednesday: Shoulders and legs
- Thursday: Follows Monday's routine
- Friday: Follows Tuesday's routine
- Saturday: Follows Wednesday's routine.

On Sunday, Hrithik rests and abstains from any physical activity and gets a full-body deep-tissue massage to ease strained muscles. After a five-day workout, it is very important that the body recovers, Satya stresses. This is essential as this recuperation is needed to heal any muscle strain or injuries that might have occurred during the workout. It also helps to build up and strengthen muscle mass. On Monday, Hrithik starts his routine again, repeating the cycle from day one. Although he doesn't spend more than two hours daily on his workouts, his sessions are so designed that they focus on burning maximum fat and building lean muscle.

Satya's Tips for Acquiring a Fit and Healthy Body

1. Eggs are the best source of protein. Make them a part of your daily diet.
2. Do cardio in the morning on an empty stomach. This will be very effective in reducing body fat and also losing abdomen fat. Hrithik has a cup of black coffee and then does cardio for an hour or forty-five minutes. After this, he works on his abs and does crunches, leg raises and hanging leg-raises.
3. Satya recommends doing weight training in the gym ideally four times a week.
4. He advises playing some kind of sports twice a week.

5. It is very important to maintain a balanced diet consisting of carbohydrates, proteins and fat throughout the year.

6. Satya believes in having two tablespoons of cow's ghee to maintain overall well-being. 'It's very good for joint lubrication.'

7. Avoid sugar altogether for six days in a week. You can have it in sweets and desserts on the seventh day which can be your cheat day.

8. Avoid too much intake of oil. If possible, try and consume not more than two teaspoons in a day.

9. Once a week, try to get a full-body deep-tissue massage. This improves blood circulation, prevents joint stiffness and eases any muscle pains.

10. Satya says that if you want to avoid putting on weight, then eat portions of rice according to the palm of your hand. So consume one bowl of mixed dal, and try to have different varieties of dal.

11. Satya recommends bulletproof coffee, which is basically one teaspoon of butter or coconut oil in your coffee; this is extremely good before workouts. This pre-workout drink gives you a lot of energy and is also good for burning fat. It increases your metabolic rate as well.

12. Try to drink hot water at least five times a day. This helps to burn fat.

13. Satya is not a party pooper. He says one can indulge once a week but make sure that you

burn the calories the very next day with some intense cardio, or else the excesses could add to your body fat.

14. A cup of hot water/green tea will help in burning fat after a heavy meal laden with calories or fat. This trick will prevent you from gaining weight. Also you can chew the skin of one-fourth of a lime to aid digestion and burn fat.

15. Satya shares a six-minute workout that is to be done in the morning on an empty stomach. This workout will keep you healthy, fit and fat-free. To be effective you must do it five times a week regularly for three months.

- Do free squats or *uthak baithak* for 1 minute. If you have a knee problem then Satya recommends ball squats, an exercise that does not put pressure on the knees.
- Do surya namaskar for a minute (for women) and push-ups for a minute (for men).
- Do jumping jacks for a minute.
- Do planks for 30 seconds the first week, 45 seconds for the second week and 1 minute the third week.
- Do side planks for 30 seconds for the first week, 45 seconds for the second week, and then 1 minute for the third week.

If these basic exercises are followed religiously for at least three months Satya says you will find yourself losing weight and staying fit. If followed throughout the year it will help in keeping your body flexible, fit and healthy.

2

Challenging All Fitness Limits: The Aamir Khan Way

Remember the suave and gentle Sanjay Singhania of *Ghajini*? After a violent encounter kills his love interest, the rich and young protagonist, who develops amnesia, transforms himself into an eight-pack wonder out to take revenge. Audiences across the country watched in amazement as a hunk emerged from the man who often portrayed sweet and playful characters.

That man is none other than Bollywood's 'Mr Perfectionist' Aamir Khan who is known to construct and deconstruct himself physically for his roles. From *Ghajini* to *3 Idiots*, *Dhoom 3* to *Dangal*, time and again, Aamir has made appearances in new physical avatars.

However, the ease with which he changes his physique almost every couple of years is no joke.

Aamir's unending dedication has elevated the art of bodybuilding to a new height. Almost every Bollywood actor these days is a fitness freak, at times displaying a muscular frame comparable to Michelangelo's *David*. But Aamir's body is almost undefinable. One year, an eight-pack muscular avenger; the next, a happy-go-lucky lean college student; the year after that, a ripped six-packed gymnast in a dual role. Who could say Sahir and Samar Khan of *Dhoom 3* were the Sanjay Singhania of *Ghajini* or the carefree Rancho of *3 Idiots*, only a few years ago? Or the overweight wrestler Mahavir Singh Phogat of *Dangal*. Earlier in the movie (but later in real life), Aamir appears on the silver screen in a completely different look of a wrestler. One wonders how a suave and fit man like him could move around with the amount of weight he had put on for *Dangal*. But he did it with elan.

Aamir Khan has achieved this versatility by sheer tenacity, a well-balanced fitness regimen and a proper diet with lots of rest.

Interestingly, in a 2010 blog post, Aamir shared the tremendous effort he put in for his continuous body transformation. This chapter will highlight the diet and exercise plans that Aamir followed to achieve the looks of his different characters.

A Structured Balanced Diet: The First Step to a Healthy Body

Most doctors and dieticians across the world stress on a balanced diet plan and discourage crash-dieting to lose weight. Aamir too ascribes to this and believes the body is not made in the gym; rather, it is the reflection of a healthy lifestyle that a person follows. One needs to put in extra effort to work on particular sets of muscles.

Amir stresses that eating less or crash-dieting is like harming yourself. It is unscientific too, as once you start depriving yourself of food, your body tends to go into starvation mode. The brain thus sends a signal to store more fat for future use. In the process, the body is also deprived of vital nutrients, which can lead to deficiency diseases. Instead, in order to aid weight loss, Aamir eats small meals frequently to increase his metabolism rate and burn more calories.

The *Ghajini* Diet

During the shooting of *Ghajini*, Aamir would eat a small meal or snack every thirty minutes. His daily calorie intake was spread across six major meals, which he was supposed to consume every two hours. In between, he needed carbohydrates to keep energy levels up, so he would eat a high-calorie fruit, like an apple or banana. Otherwise, he would opt for various vegetables, powerhouses of vital vitamins and minerals, essential for glowing skin and building immunity. Fruits and vegetables also helped him keep up his energy levels for his rigorous workouts. He had to work hard throughout the day to build that eight-pack wonder body we saw in *Ghajini*. One should remember, in this context, that any form of rigorous exercise is not possible if you are not disease-free. That's why it is essential to boost immunity to fight ailments such as common cold and viruses. That is only possible by consuming a daily dose of mixed fruits, mostly seasonal, along with green leafy vegetables, which is also why they were such an integral part of Aamir's diet.

Whenever he craved snacks, Aamir turned to brown bread sandwiches or papaya. To keep up his carbohydrate intake, he would have handmade rotis made with three kinds of cereals—wheat, jowar, bajra or other fibre-rich millets for major meals. Like multigrain toast, these multigrain rotis were big energy boosters.

To make sure he was consuming enough protein, the primary component of muscle building, Aamir would have chicken and eggs at meals on the set.

He would have one or two pieces of tandoori chicken with four egg whites or turn it into an omelette with vegetable soup. Such variety made sure it didn't become a repetitive, mundane diet routine. To keep a check on calories, every dish was cooked in just 3 tablespoons of virgin olive oil, which is light and easily digestible.

Aamir's *Ghajini* Diet Plan

Break your meals into six daily portions, and have carbohydrate-rich fruits every two hours to boost energy levels.

- The recommendation for carbohydrate intake would be multigrain rotis with fruits like apples and bananas in between meals, especially before a rigorous workout.
- If you are a non-vegetarian, your protein intake can be two to three pieces of chicken in any form along with four egg whites in any form, bhurji or omelette. Vegetarians can try out vegetable soup with salads containing protein-rich sprouts.
- Add fresh vegetables and fruits in between. Low-sugar seasonal fruits are the best. You can even try out a fruit salad if munching on whole fruits gets boring.

- If you have that craving for an evening snack, do not look for pakodas or chips, but go for healthy biscuits, brown bread sandwiches or even digestion-booster papaya cuts.
- Cook all dishes in minimal oil, preferably olive oil.

Preparing for the Dual Role in *Dhoom 3*

Dhoom 3 was indeed a challenge for Aamir Khan, despite being someone who pushes his body to the limit. For the first time on the silver screen, he played a double role of twin brothers, one of whom was autistic. Expectations were thus high from a man who had hardly ever performed action-packed sequences. He had to ride bikes, jump on trapezes and flaunt an agile acrobatic form. Such a role needed Aamir to be flexible and have fluidity of movement to portray the role of a stage gymnast. This was in sharp contrast to what the eight-pack Aamir of *Ghajini* had to do.

Dhoom 3 thus needed him to increase his basal metabolic rate (BMR), which would ensure he was full of energy to perform the high-voltage action-packed scenes as well as keep his body lean and agile by burning more calories during the day. Aamir had many meals throughout the day in small portions, to ensure his body clock kept ticking and his stomach was never empty. He also ensured he drank at least 4 litres of water each day.

While shooting, Aamir also turned to green tea. Green tea helps boost the immune system, and doctors prescribe such antioxidants to be included in daily diets. They can even fight gene mutation and keep cancer at bay.

Aamir included carbohydrates in the form of muesli during breakfast and rotis at lunch. He usually avoided carb intake during dinner to keep the meals light and healthy. Early dinners without carbohydrates seems to be one of the best diet plans and is adopted by many actors to achieve that perfect lean look. This is because one tends to be sedentary at night and carbohydrates can get stored as fat when one goes off to sleep immediately after dinner.

Once you cut down on carbs, you must include high-protein food in your meals. So Aamir's diet plan included enough egg whites, dal and grilled chicken or fish rich in essential proteins for most meals.

At times, curd was included along with fruits and sabzi to keep it vibrant. However, Aamir preferred boiled vegetables for his no-carb dinners and stuck to vegetable juices and fruits whenever he felt hungry between meals.

Aamir was usually not allowed to snack in the evening but to keep the metabolism going and feel rejuvenated, he did have rusk biscuits or cheese cubes with a steaming cup of tea.

Aamir's *Dhoom 3* Diet Plan

- Break your daily meals into six portions. Start the day with a super antioxidant like green tea to boost energy levels.
- Muesli, egg whites and seasonal fruits can make a perfect breakfast.

If you feel hungry at midday, opt for seasonal fruits or vegetable juice.

Eat the typical dal-roti-sabzi for lunch as this combination is not just healthy but also a super-light meal fortified with all nutrients. Round it off with a bowl of sour curd to boost your digestion.

Though snacking in the evening is fun, stick to just tea and a piece of light rusk or a few cheese cubes (if you're craving something salty).

- Dinner can be just a grilled chicken or boiled vegetables and fish.

Putting on Weight for *Dangal*

Just imagine if you are asked to gain 25–28 kg in just six months. It is as difficult to gain that much weight as it is to shed it. *Dangal* director Nitesh Tewari did give Aamir the option of wearing a bodysuit to camouflage his *Dhoom 3* six-pack abs.

But Aamir took the harder route. He gained the extra weight first, shot the larger part of the movie as an overweight wrestler, and then shed that extra flab for the other half of the movie. This transformation needed an extremely well-monitored diet plan and indeed a lot of determination.

To go from fat (gaining almost 28 kg in six months) to fit, Aamir followed a strict diet plan under the supervision of Dr Vinod Dhurander. He first turned vegan, giving up milk and milk products completely. Vegan diets have, in recent years, taken Hollywood by storm. Hollywood heart-throb Natalie Portman, while explaining why she switched from a vegetarian diet to a vegan diet, made it clear it was not just to show solidarity with animals by not using dairy products, but also to avoid factory-made dairy products. In 2011, when she was pregnant, she did go back to consuming meat and milk, but returned to a vegan diet after childbirth.

Not eating meat also helped Aamir imbibe the role more as Mahavir Phogat was a vegetarian.

In Aamir's own words, 'Putting on weight was fun as I could eat and drink whatever I wanted. I had a ball, I have to say, but it was uncomfortable.' Getting used to the extra weight is indeed a challenge for anyone who has been as fit as Aamir. And if you are into a sport like wrestling, then it becomes even more difficult. Aamir's wrestling training was affected as he had to carry the extra flab and was unable to move fast. Excess weight can put pressure on the heart and lungs, leading to heavy breathing when you run, walk briskly or jump, like one needs to in wrestling.

There were times when Aamir thought his decision to gain the weight first and then go on to lose it was not correct. But he showed enough courage to carry around 97 kg and 38 per cent body fat. He ate about 1800–2500 calories a day to pile on the extra weight. This was the opposite of his diet philosophy: 'Diet is number one in changing your body. It doesn't matter how much you exercise—if your diet isn't right, the results won't show.'

However, the man who oversaw Aamir Khan's magical transformation, breaking all myths of fit and flab, believes everyone should go by a specific requirement and not follow others blindly. Dr Nikhil Dhurandar, professor at the Department of Nutrition at Texas Tech University and former president of the Obesity Society, knew Aamir had to simultaneously lose body fat and gain big muscles, something that is very difficult to achieve. Hence, he developed a dietary sheet for the actor, keeping in mind his likes and dislikes and changed the plan regularly to make it exciting. The result was stupendous, from an overweight obese man to a Greek god flaunting those perfect pectorals!

If you're aiming for similar results, ensure your diet plan is safe. Slow and gradual weight gain or loss does not shock the system.

The diet chart should not, at any point, be unbalanced or overloaded with proteins, nor should essential nutrients like minerals and vitamins be ignored. Aamir's *Dangal* diet, when he had to shed the weight, included small frequent meals with in-between snacks of fruits and vegetable juices.

A Peek into Aamir Khan's *Dangal* Dietary Sheet

Every day at dawn (around 4 a.m.), Aamir was given one whole egg omelette with a sprinkle of onions, tomato, coriander leaves and green chillies. This was done to boost the metabolism for the whole day.

- He used to start off his day with one level scoop of protein shake at around 6 a.m.
- Two hours later, he would switch to eating fruits (around 150 g). High-calorie fruits like banana were avoided in the morning.

- At around 10 a.m., he was given 50 g of poha with chopped onions, tomatoes and green chillies to make it tasty.
- A quick pre-lunch snack included one slice of bread and 100 g of tuna.
- Two hours later, he had a proper lunch that included 50 g rice, two kinds of vegetable dishes (100 g each), 15 g of dal and 200 g of low-fat curd.
- At 4 p.m. he ate fruits as snacks (except banana).
- Around 6 p.m., he was again allowed to eat a slice of brown bread with any fish, like tuna.
- Dinner had to be finished by 7 p.m. with almost the same menu as lunch.
- All meals for the day were cooked in a meagre 5 teaspoons of oil.
- He was allowed to indulge in a cup of black tea without sugar/milk.

As Fit as Aamir

Aamir Khan has defied age at times and pushed his body to the limit where even pain resulting from muscle overwork did not deter him. After all, how many people can painstakingly work out for four hours a day, every day?

But perfectionist Aamir has never left any stone unturned to achieve unimaginable goals. His trainer, Satyajit Chaurasia, has always praised him for his tenacity and willpower. The stomach crunches Aamir had to do for *Dhoom 3* were extremely painful initially, but he was so dedicated to his strict fitness regimen that he did not miss a single day at the gym while shooting for the film. He kept up the crunches for three months at a stretch. Once those muscles are regularly exercised, the tension releases and they fall into place, and the pain also subsides.

Aamir has always spoken of a three-point approach towards building these muscles and making them look amazing on-screen: a balanced diet, rigorous exercise and enough sleep. The actor has repeatedly said in interviews that sleep is as important to him as exercise. He advises those who are interested in building muscles and sculpting their body to not underestimate the power of resting. While shooting for *Ghajini*, Aamir used to sleep for at least eight hours every night.

Aamir's Regular Gym Routine

Aamir is 5 feet 6 inches tall and weighs about 74 kg on average. His routine workout involves stretching exercises with dumb-bells, meditation and yoga. Here's a look at his weekly exercise plan:

- Aamir has kept Monday for toning up his chest. According to him the best exercises for the chest are bench presses, incline dumb-bell presses, decline presses, dumb-bell flyes and dumb-bell pull-overs. Press exercises are extremely effective in producing a chiselled chest, exactly what Aamir Khan needed for his role in *Dhoom 3*. The upper and middle chest is best stimulated by bench-press exercises.

- It is as important to work out the shoulders as the chest, which is why Aamir replaces the chest exercises with shoulder exercises on Tuesday. Shoulders comprise three major muscles known as deltoids, and it is very important to develop all three. If one of the muscles is underdeveloped, the whole shoulder starts paining. Since chest exercises do not take care of the lateral and posterior deltoids, one has to dedicate one day to focus on these muscles of the shoulder region. Shoulder exercises should be balanced in such a way that both shoulders look the same. Aamir makes sure to do military presses, front shoulder-presses, sheet dumb-bell presses, shoulder presses, bent-over lateral presses and upright rows.

- Amir Khan's back exercises on Wednesdays include T-bar rows, seated cable rows, lat pull-down fronts, fronted chin-ups, one-arm dumb-bell rows and dead-lifts. Back exercises are a group of combined exercises, and Aamir goes for the perfect balance as wrong exercise can lead to lower-back pain. Back muscles are as important as the chest muscles because the weight of almost the entire body and arms rests on the back.

- Thursdays and Fridays are for bicep- and tricep-muscle development. Aamir alternates barbell curls, dumb-bell curls, preacher curls, concentration curls, wrist curls and reverse curls. For triceps, a mix of presses and kickbacks are most effective. The ones that Aamir does are short-grip triceps presses, rope pull-downs, cable lying triceps extensions, dumb-bell kickbacks and dips behind the back.

- Aamir needed well-toned and sturdy legs for the role of a gymnast in *Dhoom 3* as well as for *Ghajini*. Leg exercises are very intense and hence Aamir prefers to keep them for the last day of the week, after which he takes a break for a day. Saturdays are for squats, lunges, leg curls, leg extensions and seated toe-raises for the calves.

- A flat and taut abdomen is every man's dream. He spends time doing decline crunches, dumb-bell side bends, crossover crunches, hanging leg-raises and seated knee-ups (done on an ab cruncher) on Mondays, Wednesdays and Fridays to make sure he has a strong core and maintains those abs.

In case you plan to attempt a similar routine or build your own workout using Aamir's as inspiration, please keep in mind the level of your fitness, and the correct form and posture required for each exercise. Try to seek help from a trainer who can guide you about these exercises.

How Aamir Khan Learnt Swimming

In Reema Kagti's 2012 suspense thriller, *Talaash*, Aamir Khan played the role of Inspector Shekhawat, a cop trying to come to terms with his son's death and a failing marriage, while also investigating a high-profile death.

Aamir needed to shoot an underwater sequence in the film but he had never learnt swimming. Aamir had no clue how to do an underwater sequence without being a swimmer. But being a hardcore professional, he refused to have a stunt double, wanting to do the whole underwater sequence himself. That meant he needed to learn deepwater or underwater swimming, which can be more challenging than regular swimming.

It is difficult to take up swimming as an adult, but Aamir's dedication towards anything he does helped to sail him through. So much so that the director had to admit she was impressed with Aamir's swimming skills and the entire crew was surprised as to how the actor had picked up swimming so easily.

He learnt primary swimming from Micky Mehta. And his trainer, David Clark Salo (popularly known as Dave), helped him learn progressive underwater swimming. Aamir says, 'David helped me prepare for the underwater sequence with breathing exercises to increase my lung power so that I could stay underwater longer.'

Aamir's Workout Regimen for His Eight-pack Abs in *Ghajini*

Sporting an eight-pack in *Ghajini* required a tremendous amount of effort. Usually Bollywood heroes flaunt a six-pack abdomen in most movies, but Aamir wanted to go a step further. This led to an extremely gruelling and hectic exercise routine for him. For almost thirteen months, he worked day and night to bring about that near-impossible look in the action-packed murder mystery.

Aamir sweated out for three hours a day, six days a week, for thirteen months non-stop. His workout schedule was divided into ten minutes of stretching, forty minutes of abs and side exercises and then weight training.

For the special abs workout to achieve an eight-pack, he followed a separate routine of decline crunches, dumb-bell side bends, crossover crunches, hanging leg-raise and seated knee-up.

He also slept for a minimum of eight hours and adhered to the diet plan mentioned earlier.

A Day-to-day Look at Aamir's *Ghajini* Workouts

Monday
- 4 sets of barbell bench-presses of 10–12 repeats
- 4 sets of incline barbell bench-presses of 10–12 reps
- 4 sets of decline barbell bench-presses of 12 reps
- 4 sets of dumb-bell flyes of 12–15 reps
- 4 sets of dumb-bell pull-overs of 12–15 reps
- 4 sets of cable press-downs of 10–12 reps
- 4 sets of triceps extensions of 10–12 reps
- 4 sets of one-arm triceps extensions of 8–10 reps
- 4 sets of triceps clips of 10–15 reps

Tuesday
- 4 sets of dumb-bell presses of 12–15 reps
- 4 sets of front shoulder-presses of 10–12 reps
- 4 sets of bent-over shoulder-raises of 10–12 reps
- 4 sets of dumb-bell shrugs of 12 reps
- 4 sets of lateral dumb-bell raises of 12–15 reps
- 4 sets of barbell military-presses of 12–15 reps

Wednesday
- 4 sets of lateral pull-downs of 12–15 reps
- 4 sets of cable seated rows of 12–15 reps
- 4 sets of one-arm dumb-bell rows of 10–12 reps
- 4 sets of T-bar rows of 10–15 reps
- 4 sets of lateral dumb-bell curls of 12–15 reps
- 4 sets of preacher curls of 12–15 reps

- 4 sets of lateral concentration-curls of 12–15 reps
- 4 sets of barbell curls of 12–15 reps
- 4 sets of wrist curls of 12–15 reps

Thursday
- 4 sets of seated leg-tucks of 12–15 reps
- 4 sets of back extensions of 10–12 reps
- 4 sets of vertical bench-crunches of 10–12 reps
- 4 sets of hanging leg-raises of 10–15 reps
- 4 sets of crunches with a stability ball of 12–15 reps
- 4 sets of crossover crunches of 12–15 reps
- 4 sets of seated knee-ups of 10–12 reps

Friday
- 4 sets of barbell squats of 12–15 reps
- 4 sets of barbell lunges of 10–12 reps
- 4 sets of leg-press machine of 10–15 reps
- 4 sets of leg-curl machine of 10–15 reps
- 4 sets of standing calf-raises of 12–15 reps
- 4 sets of seated toe-raises for calves of 12–15 reps

Saturday and Sunday
- Rest and recovery

Aamir's Gruelling Routine to Achieve the Flexible Body of a Gymnast in *Dhoom* 3

To get a gymnast's body at the age of fifty, Aamir Khan needed to be fit and flexible. For hours, he trained in martial arts apart from swimming daily for more than an hour. He primarily concentrated on basic stretching exercises but also made sure that targeted muscles were rubbed to create warmth and increase blood flow to the area. A dedicated and hard-working man, Aamir achieved that agile figure in just four months.

Gerald Zarcilla, who is an acrobat himself, was one of Aamir's fitness trainers for *Dhoom 3* over those four months. In an interview, Zarcilla said, 'When I first met Aamir, he had a physique similar to his *3 Idiots* days—very lean and not what you would expect out of an action hero or a gymnast.'[1] He designed special training schedules for Aamir and included high-intensity interval training cardio exercises. The cardio intervals included boxing and low- and high-impact aerobic exercises. Resistance training was also done with gymnastics to help Aamir shoot some of the song sequences where he had to hang from trapeze ropes. Gymnastic exercises included rolling V-sits, which are great for toning the body and building up core strength.

Aamir Khan has admitted several times that *Dhoom 3* was his toughest movie so far. In his words, 'I have never played anything like this before. Every film is challenging, but this was a tough role. I am playing a gymnast in the film. I also went for circus training for the film. There was a lot of hard work followed by [a] strict diet.'[2]

For *Dhoom 3*, Aamir Khan followed a similar exercise regimen as he does at the gym every day. But his trainers added a twist. More importance was given to his back muscles, biceps, triceps, chest and shoulders. He took complete rest on Saturdays and Sundays and maintained a five-day-a-week gym routine.

He also added a couple of new crunches for his abdominal/core workout, which included seated leg-tucks, back extensions, vertical bench-crunches, hanging leg-raises and crunches with stability ball. For triceps, he added cable press-downs, one-arm tricep extensions and triceps dips, with barbell bench-presses, incline barbell bench-presses, decline barbell bench-presses and dumb-bell flyes. The number of sets and reps he would do was similar to the routine followed for *Ghajini*.

Dangal

Dangal was a different challenge compared to *Dhoom 3* as Aamir had to move around with more than 90 kg and even train himself for the wrestling sessions. For the later part of the movie, Aamir trained in Arizona and took to outdoor activities like trekking, swimming, tennis and cycling, which automatically reduce weight and increase his BMR. These sports also helped tone the muscles.

Yoga and Aamir Khan

Aamir has always turned to yoga whenever he has needed to make his mind and body work in tandem. Yoga in various forms has made inroads into lives of Bollywood and Hollywood stars over the years. A peaceful mind is the gateway to a healthy body. Aamir practises yoga and meditation every time he has to calm his nerves. He practises pranayama too, which helps him concentrate and focus on his skills.

Conclusion

Anyone wishing to flaunt an ever-changing physique like Aamir must push themselves to extremes as he does. But training hard isn't sufficient. As Aamir has always put it, one must ensure a minimum eight hours of sleep, proper diet and discipline. Everything takes time, nothing happens overnight.

Aamir is so serious and sincere about his workouts and diet that he meticulously counts every calorie he consumes and how much he burns daily. He not only works out at the gym, he also loves to play various sports to avoid boredom. No wonder Aamir is Aamir!

3

Priyanka Chopra: Bold and Beautiful

Bollywood Background

Time magazine named her one of the 100 most influential people in the world in 2016. She has received numerous awards, including a National Film Award and five Filmfare Awards. In 2016, the Indian government conferred the Padma Shri, the fourth-highest civilian award upon her. She is also one of the highest-paid actresses in the country.

Unstoppable, undeniably beautiful and unanimously popular, Priyanka Chopra is definitely on top of her game.

She first made her mark when she became Miss World in 2000. Since then, she has proved herself a force to reckon with.

She made her Bollywood debut in *The Hero: Love Story of a Spy* (2003). In 2004, she played a negative character in the thriller *Aitraaz* and received critical acclaim for the role. She went on to star in highly successful commercial ventures like *Don* and *Krrish* opposite superstars like Shah Rukh Khan and Hrithik Roshan respectively, and thus established herself in the top league of actresses.

Fashion (2008) won her the Filmfare and National Film Award for best actress. An extremely versatile and gifted actress, she has not been afraid to try her hand at playing unconventional roles that most popular actresses would have refused. She gained recognition for her roles in *7 Khoon Maaf* (2011), *Barfi* (2012), *Mary Kom* (2014), *Dil Dhadakne Do* (2015) and *Bajirao Mastani* (2016). Having done some exemplary work in Bollywood, she has moved to Los Angeles and now New York to pursue her career as a TV star, in the highly popular thriller series *Quantico*. Here she plays the action-packed role of undercover agent Alex Parrish.

Her philanthropic work is also phenomenal. She has worked with UNICEF for the last ten years and was appointed the national and global UNICEF goodwill ambassador for child rights in 2010 and 2016 respectively. In addition to this, she promotes various causes such as environment, health, education, women's rights and is very supportive and vocal about gender equality and feminism.

But her list of laurels doesn't stop there. As a recording artist she has released three singles. Apart from being a talented actress, she's also an excellent dancer, as is evident from her films. So how does this fabulously gifted and busy actress keep herself looking so fit?

Fit and Fabulous

Priyanka is a strong proponent of yoga, which is highly recommended by fitness trainers these days because of its numerous health benefits. Very good for increased muscle strength and tone, it helps perfect your posture. Yoga also prevents cartilage and joint breakdown because each time you practise it, you take your joints through their full range of motion. This prevents degenerative arthritis by activating areas of the cartilage that aren't normally used. It can help protect your spine if you practise a well-rounded number of asanas that have plenty of backbends, forward bends and twists to keep your disks supple. This vastly improves flexibility.

In fact, Samir Jaura, who trained Priyanka for the movie *Mary Kom*, said he is yet to see someone as flexible as her. Priyanka credits her flexibility and toned physique to yoga.

Yoga asanas, pranayama and meditation are part of her daily fitness routine. Priyanka also turns to yoga as it is a great stress-buster, keeping her calm and relaxed in her busy and hectic schedule. Yoga relaxes the system because it encourages you to relax, slow your breath and focus on the present, thus shifting the balance from the sympathetic nervous system (or the fight or flight response) to the parasympathetic nervous system. The latter lowers breathing and the heart rate, decreases blood pressure and increases blood flow to the intestines and reproductive organs. The right asanas, pranayama and meditation can also stimulate it to help you sleep deeper and boost your immune system's functionality.

Priyanka also credits yoga for her toned body and high stamina. The tree pose, half lord of the fishes pose and warrior pose are some of the asanas she incorporates into her daily routine.

Priyanka once confided in Samir who wanted to train her more intensely for *Don* that she is not a gym freak but does work out regularly to keep her body toned and fit. She didn't want to shrink by two or three sizes though. She has always maintained she is against drastic weight loss and avoids looking too skinny. Her preference tends to a routine to maintain her weight at an optimum level she feels comfortable with. Priyanka works out for four days a week for an hour in the gym. Her routine in the gym looks like this:

- Running on the treadmill for about 15 minutes
- Push-ups and reverse lunges

- 20–25 reverse crunches and 20–25 bench jumps
- 20–25 bicep curls with light weights
- 60-second planks.

Priyanka prefers resistance training over weight training as it increases the body's strength and endurance levels. She also does running and takes spin classes from time to time.

For ideal results, fitness experts like Nawaz Modi Singhania recommend a combination of cardio and yoga: three to four days of cardio with two to three days of yoga each week is a killer combo. The two schools of fitness training complement each other, according to Nawaz. One should also keep a day for resting. Clearly, this has worked well for Priyanka.

She also maintains a regular workout routine that is a combination of the two. She does not believe in overdoing it at the gym just so that she can maintain her curvaceous figure.

Punjabi *Kudi* at Heart

Priyanka confesses that she is a typical Punjabi kudi and loves to indulge in home-cooked Punjabi food and tandoori dishes. She's also quite lucky because in spite of indulging regularly, she doesn't put on weight. The reason is she has a high metabolism. So, on weekends she gives in to her cravings for sweet temptations, such as cakes and chocolates.

On regular days, Priyanka makes it a point to eat small meals every two hours. This keeps her metabolic rate high and prevents her from overeating in one single meal.

Her meal plan for a day usually looks like this:

- Breakfast: Two egg whites/oatmeal with a glass of skimmed milk.
- Lunch: Two rotis with a bowl of dal and plenty of salad and veggies.
- Evening snack: Turkey sandwich/a bowl of sprout salad.
- Dinner: A bowl of soup followed by grilled chicken/fish along with some sautéed veggies.
- She drinks plenty of water throughout the day, and prefers fruit juices over aerated drinks. Coconut water with some nuts every couple of hours keeps her active and energized.

Priyanka's Power-packed Punches: The *Mary Kom* Way

Samir Jaura, who trained Priyanka for the film, says that, surprisingly, Priyanka had had no experience with weight training before this. 'So the training for *Mary Kom* was a shock to her system. And that is why her body responded so well. But of course she was fit and flexible, else she would have been unable to undergo the rigorous workouts I put her through.'

Samir says this about Priyanka's abhorrence for gruelling workouts, 'I trained her for *Don 2*. And she hated me for the workout sessions I put her through, as she felt they were very painful!' But soon the two were working together again on a film that demanded every ounce of Priyanka's physical commitment. For five to six months, Samir put her through some torturous workouts.

Along with working out with Samir in the evening for the look the script required, Priyanka trained with a boxer in the mornings.

Samir points out that although the role necessitated the look of a boxer: 'My brief was to not make her look too bulky or muscular.'

The trainer read and researched about Mary Kom's life and way of training. He also studied her body language, which he in turn taught Priyanka for her role. But as he points out, 'It was not possible for Priyanka to pick up all aspects of Mary Kom's training. That would have been impossible as she is after all an actress and not an Olympian boxer with fifteen years of training experience behind her.'

Mary Kom starts her day by running a distance of 14 km every day. She does stretching exercises and shadow-boxing after that. In the evenings, Mary goes to the gym, where she does strength-training exercises and practises her boxing in the ring. An important part of Mary's workout is to maintain brain and eye coordination for speed and power, which are the most important aspects of the sport. Lastly, she cools off with a short run after her strenuous training session.

The following are some of the basic exercises that were incorporated into Priyanka's training regimen, and can be beneficial for anyone if done in conjunction with each other. They will not only help achieve the level of fitness that Priyanka did, but also improve speed, muscle tone, stamina and agility:

- Jump rope: It's a fantastic way to get your muscles ready and increase your stamina. Samir recommends that you start with 50 counts and then increase it by 10 jumps every week.
- Shadow-boxing: It's the action of practising your punches against an imaginary opponent. This workout helps the boxer speed up the hand and leg movements. It also increases flexibility and alertness. Samir recommends doing this for 30 minutes in a day.

- Stretches: Do at least 3 stretching exercises that will help increase your flexibility. Priyanka includes the warrior pose, which is good for flexibility of the legs and arms. Then the 'half lord of the fishes' pose is good for the flexibility of the hips and relieves back problems. The tree pose makes the arms more flexible and balances the body.
- Strength-building exercises: Strength training does more than just make you strong. Its additional benefits include higher bone density, stronger joints, improved balance and stability, more stamina and better posture. Samir recommends 10 burpees, 10 push-ups, 10 pull-ups, 10 barbell squats, 10 reverse crunches, 10 kettlebell swings and 10 tricep dips in a day.

Samir mentions that as Priyanka had no formal training with lifting weights and other strength-training exercises, her body responded very well to the workouts. He says, 'If your body gets used to a particular workout or form of training then it is unlikely to show any particularly great result. But if you keep changing your workouts and challenge your body in different ways then you are likely to see noticeable results. That's why Priyanka's body started to look really amazing in a short period of time.'

Samir is full of praise for her focus and single-mindedness. 'During her training for the film, PC lost her father. But it was so commendable and professional of her that she came back to shoot in six days flat. She did not keep the rest of the unit waiting for her. I admire her dedication and discipline.'

To do justice to the biopic of Mary Kom and look the part, Priyanka's training programme also included a lot of functional training, high-rep training to improve her stamina, and core workouts and stretching before and after workouts to enhance flexibility. Priyanka trained for four and a half months before the shoot and two months during the shoot.

She underwent a high-intensity circuit training that lasted for about twelve weeks.

Needless to say, Priyanka who hates any formal high-intensity training gave it her all and performed to the best of her physical abilities. She displayed tremendous tenacity and staying power.

One day while training, Priyanka turned to Samir and said, 'Samir, I'm going to win the National Award for this film.' And that's exactly what she did.

Priyanka's 12-week Workout Schedule (6 Days a Week)

Weeks 1 and 2
Basic stretching, spot jogging, treadmill (20 minutes), jump rope (30 reps), burpees (10 reps), mountain

climbers (10 reps), squats (10 reps), high knees (20 reps), side bends (40 reps), crunches (20 reps). 1-minute rest. Repeat 5 times. Treadmill (20 minutes).

Weeks 3 and 4

Basic stretching, spot jogging and treadmill (20 minutes), jump rope (50 reps), burpees (10 reps), squats (15 reps), lunges (20 reps), push-ups (10 reps), leg raises (10 reps), side bends (40 reps), mountain climbers (40 reps). 1-minute rest. Repeat this 5 times. Treadmill (20 minutes).

Weeks 5 and 6

Basic stretching, spot jogging, treadmill (20 minutes), squats (15 reps), lunges (20 reps), push-ups (15 reps), pull-ups (10 reps), shoulder presses with bands (10 reps), sit-ups (25 reps), leg raises (25 reps), rotations (15 reps). 1-minute rest. Repeat this 5 times. Treadmill (20 minutes).

Weeks 7 and 8

Basic stretching, spot jogging, treadmill (20 minutes), squats (15 reps), lunges (20 reps), push-ups (15 reps), pull-ups (10 reps), shoulder presses with bands (15 reps), sit-ups (25 reps), leg raises (25 reps), rotations (15 reps). 1-minute rest. Repeat this 6 times. Treadmill (20 minutes).

Weeks 9 and 10
Basic stretching, running (20 minutes), lunges (5 sets, 15 reps), front lat pull-downs (5 sets, 15 reps), incline presses (5 sets, 15 reps), front presses (5 times, 15 reps), concentration curls (4 sets, times 12 reps), tricep extension with dumb-bells (4 sets, 12 reps), side bends (4 sets, 100 reps), crunches (4 sets, 100 reps), leg raises (4 sets, 100 reps), treadmill (20 minutes).

Weeks 11 and 12
Basic stretching, running (20 minutes), lunges (5 sets, 15 reps), front lat pull-downs (5 sets, 15 reps), incline presses (5 sets, 15 reps), front presses (5 times, 15 reps), concentration curls (4 sets, 12 reps), tricep extension with dumb-bells (4 sets, 12 reps), side bends (4 sets, 100 reps), crunches (4 sets, 100 reps), leg raises (4 sets, 100 reps).

Diet for *Mary Kom*

Samir reveals, 'Before I met her for the film, Priyanka was not following any particular diet plan. She was quite flexible regarding her eating habits. She wouldn't think twice about eating a samosa or pastry. But after shooting for this film she became conscious of her eating habits.'

The actual boxer or Mary Kom follows a diet that contains 40–55 per cent complex carbohydrates for fulfilling her energy requirements throughout the day. She also makes sure to incorporate 10 per cent healthy fats for vitamin and mineral absorption, 40 per cent lean proteins for strength and muscle repair, and plenty of fluids and electrolytes for hydration and stamina. Thus, a basic diet plan followed by a boxer for a healthy and strong body would comprise:

- Breakfast: Fruits, a glass of milk or protein shake, cereals, oatmeal or wholewheat bread with any organic cheese. Water.
- Snacks: Carrots, cucumber slices, an apple or a banana as well as a protein shake.
- Lunch: One serving of meat or fish, boiled vegetables with cheese or a raw vegetable salad. A bowl of brown or white steamed rice. A cup of plain or green tea.
- Evening snack: A protein shake or any home-made fruit juice and a bowl of fat-free yogurt.
- Dinner: A bowl of salad, one serving of meat, chicken or fish along with steamed rice.
- Last snack: A glass of milk and a fruit.
- Sports persons who follow such rigorous routines make sure to stay well hydrated at all times and eliminate junk food completely from their diet.
- While planning the diet, Samir kept in mind that it would have to provide enough energy for her

strenuous workouts, and would need to have the necessary bodybuilding proteins and plenty of fluids.

- Priyanka's diet was broken into five to six meals a day with a three-hour gap between each meal.
- Breakfast: 3 to 4 egg whites/ 1 bowl of oatmeal with skimmed milk and raisins, walnuts and almonds
- Midday snack: A fruit and a protein shake
- Lunch: A bowl of sautéed veggies (spinach, bell peppers, mushrooms, beans and broccoli)
- Evening snack: Fruits and 1 glass of green coconut water
- Dinner: Grilled fish (100 to 150 g) and a bowl of veggies.

Priyanka prefers spicy food but as Samir had put her on a bland diet with minimal salt intake, she would use a tiny bit of Tabasco sauce from time to time to spice up the food. Salt was practically eliminated from her diet to prevent bloating and water retention, and only two tablespoons of olive oil were used throughout the day to prepare Priyanka's meals.

Samir praises Priyanka's discipline and determination in following the diet as she is not used to eating such bland and tasteless food.

Priyanka's Fitness Tips

1. Drink the required amount of fluids to keep your body hydrated during workouts.
2. Eat more home-cooked food. Make sure you have a balanced diet with lots of veggies and fruits for fibre, proteins and carbs.
3. Avoid oily and deep-fried foods.
4. Don't suppress your cravings totally. Indulge once a week if you are not prone to weight gain.
5. Practise yoga as it is excellent for the body and the mind.

Priyanka has proved time and again that her fitness mantras work for her, whether through her versatile roles in Bollywood or while working her way up to international fame and stardom in Hollywood through *Quantico* and *Baywatch*.

By making a niche for herself in Hollywood, Priyanka has proved that she is feisty, fearless and fabulously talented. She has moved out of the comfort zone of Bollywood and into the international arena, where she is making a name for herself amongst other international celebrities.

4

Varun: Dhawan and Only

In 2012, a romantic comedy drama, directed by Karan Johar was released from the stables of Dharma Productions in collaboration with Shah Rukh Khan's Red Chillies Entertainment. The movie *Student of the Year* featured newcomers Siddharth Malhotra, Varun Dhawan and Alia Bhatt in the lead roles and went on to become one of the highest-grossing Bollywood blockbusters of 2012. The success of the movie propelled the three new actors into stardom. Siddharth Malhotra came from outside the film fraternity but Varun Dhawan, a scion of the Dhawan family—his father, the director David, and uncle and yesteryear actor Anil, have been part of the Bollywood entertainment fraternity for more than four decades now—caught the public's attention with his arrival.

Veni, vidi, vici—he came, he saw, he conquered. Recipient of the Lions Gold Award and Stardust

Award for best male debut, Varun was a sensation and became an idol for millennials all over the country.

Born on 24 April 1987 to film director David and Karuna Dhawan, Varun was always a gifted student. He studied business management at the Nottingham Trent University before returning to work as an assistant director in Karan Johar's 2010 drama, *My Name Is Khan*

After *Student of the Year*, Dhawan established himself in Bollywood by starring in the romantic movie *Humpty Sharma Ki Dulhania* (2014) and *ABCD 2* (2015), both of which grossed over Rs 1 billion worldwide. He then garnered a nomination for the Filmfare Award for best actor for portraying an avenger in the crime thriller *Badlapur* (2015). Dhawan subsequently starred in the action drama *Dilwale* (2015), the crime drama *Dishoom* (2016), and the romantic comedy *Badrinath Ki Dulhania* (2017). *Dilwale* went on to become one of the highest-grossing Bollywood films. Varun had a different look in each of these movies and brought his exceptional sense of comic timing to every role. He excelled at even the thriller sequences, allowing his great body to do all the talking. For example, in *Main Tera Hero,* Varun turned even fight sequences into humorous banter. His six-pack body is not a trope by itself, but rather part and parcel of his complete package. His muscular frame is very much a part of his personality that blends well with the characters he portrays on-screen.

How Varun's Physique Is Different from Other Bollywood Actors

Varun's charming looks and chiselled physique have given him an edge over many other actors of his generation. He is a great dancer with an extremely agile and flexible body, and to maintain that he hits the gym regularly. Since childhood, Hollywood hunks Sylvester Stallone and Arnold Schwarzenegger have been his ultimate heroes, and he has always particularly wished to have the macho man-machine physique of Stallone. He even uploaded a picture of the two on Instagram saying, 'Arnold and Stallone. One at the age of seventy and the other at sixty-nine. Inspiring us all even now.' It was Stallone's Rocky franchise that struck a chord with young Dhawan and led him to have a deep interest in films.

Varun has always been a sports enthusiast. He was an athlete in his schooldays and worked hard at an early age to improve his fitness and stamina. He was a very good swimmer all through his student days. Even now, he always finds time to swim for at least half an hour despite a busy schedule. Varun is also good at cricket and squash and is often seen playing the two to improve his agility and endurance. In his own words: 'I have come to realize that filling your day with various activities keeps your weight in place. I rely on the Nike Fuel Band that tracks how much, how often, and how intensely you move. If you need abs, workouts are necessary because any sport cuts down the fat. Sports are great for the mind too and keep it active.'[1] He could not be more right in this respect. Team sports in particular are good for inculcating good habits like accountability, dedication and leadership. Fighting for a common goal with a host of other players, coaches, managers and community members teaches you how to build synergy and effectively communicate the best way to solve problems. This helps Varun solve any problem he encounters at work, at home, or on the sets. Thus, playing a sport is a winning combination for Dhawan.

What Fitness Means to Varun

With sculpted arms, toned legs and washboard abs, Varun is the new fitness icon. However, his outlook on fitness is not conventional. Rather, over the years, his fitness mantra has become more philosophical and down-to-earth.

For Varun, fitness is not about displaying beefy muscles and a well-toned body, but rather a state of mind. In other words, he aims to sculpt his body in a manner that is in harmony both physically and mentally. Varun defines an ideal body as one that has enough stamina to perform daily activities smoothly, develop a better and stronger immunity and which, at the same time, is ready for tough tasks and challenges. He believes concentrating solely on building muscles tends to make the body rigid and this can impede fast and varied dance moves, which he is so famous for.

His balanced training regimen helps him maintain a sculpted physique and flexibility. The fluidity of his movement lends a certain gracefulness to every twist and turn of the limbs and the torso. Varun's lean physique helps him attain his desired goal with ease. However, it does not mean he puts in less effort.

Varun's Fitness Guru

Varun exercises under the famed celebrity fitness guru Prashant Sawant, winner of Men's Health Best Personal Trainer in India Award 2014. Sawant is also the personal trainer of superstars like Shah Rukh Khan and Ajay Devgn. He took Varun under his wing from the time the young actor set his foot in the industry.

Varun is very disciplined and self-motivated when it comes to workouts. He is a powerhouse of energy, and Sawant sees to it that the strict exercise regimen does not get monotonous and boring for his young disciple. So, from time to time Sawant devises surprise tasks and makes his training sessions interesting and challenging. This motivates Varun to hit the gym even after a tiring and busy outdoor session. He is keen to go for his workouts, and looks forward to stretch his limits and perform the tasks Sawant puts him through.

Another tactic that Sawant uses to motivate Varun is, as he says, 'I send him pictures of his best-looking body and ask him if what he is now matches with it, and he is like, "Oh! I am coming right now to the gym."'

However, on the few rare days when Varun confesses he is dead tired, Sawant doesn't push him and lets him off the hook without much fuss because he knows that rest days are an essential part of training. While it may seem like one is slacking and make you worry that you won't build strength or increase speed or lose weight, time off allows the body and mind to fully recover and grow. Never taking a day off sets the body up for a breakdown. One becomes more susceptible to severe muscle soreness, a suppressed immune system, improper sleep, a decrease in strength and performance, and injury. Rest days also benefit one's mind: Scheduling a mandatory break from training helps Varun rejuvenate and be excited to jump back into his programme.

In one of his interviews to *Stardust*, Sawant confided, 'When Varun first came to me for *Student of the Year*, he already had a structure in place, but there was something lacking which made him get lost in the crowd. He needed an edge.' Sawant's wife, Maya, a sports nutritionist, worked in tandem with her husband to help Varun plan his daily diet.

Varun also trains under renowned fitness coach and Pilates trainer Namrata Purohit. 'Varun works out for about one and a half hours, four to six times a week, depending on his schedule. He does a mix of Pilates and weight training, and works on strengthening his body as well as on agility, flexibility, balance and stability,'[2] says Purohit.

Pilates sessions have made him more flexible, lean, and improved his balance. He has become a lot stronger and is also able to cope better with injuries and prevent them.

Varun's Regular Workout Sessions

He usually starts his workout session with simple warm-up exercises for ten to fifteen minutes, alternating between jogging and swimming. He then moves on to cardio and heavy-weights training. Warm-up exercises are vital for preparing the body and setting the pace for heavy exercises later as they increase the heart rate, activate the muscles and prevent sudden injuries during a heavy workout. Varun realized this when he injured his hip bone during an action sequence while shooting for *Main Tera Hero*; he blamed not warming up before the shot for that incident.

Varun's regular workout comprises martial training and cardio workouts. He also practises light weightlifting which is an essential part of forming a sculpted physique. He makes sure that his weights never go beyond 25–30 kg. He alters the weights from light to hefty and then hefty to light. This prevents his weight loss from plateauing.

His exercise regimen includes plenty of stretching exercises, targeted to improve the shoulder and chest area. He advises, 'While doing stretching postures of yoga, make sure that you perform reverse exercise as well for every stretching exercise done; else, you are likely to get [a] painful back.'[3]

Varun's gym training focuses on perfecting and sculpting individual body parts. On the first day of the week, he begins with chest and triceps. For this, he needs 3–4 warm-up sets followed by 3–4 incline dumb-bell presses, four working sets of 8–20 reps, 3 working sets of incline dumb-bell flyes of 8–10 reps, machine bench-press warm-up sets, followed by reverse-grip tricep push-downs (straight bar) as well as seated triceps-presses.

On the second day, he concentrates on shoulders. For this, he does upright cable row, a multi-joint movement, unlike raises, which is considered more of a finesse move. This makes upright rows the perfect transitional move in the middle of one's delt workout, front barbell-raise, cable front raise, machine shoulder-presses, leaning dumb-bell lateral raise, cable rear-delt fly, the Arnold dumb-bell press (research shows it's the most effective exercise you can do to build anterior-deltoid strength and it also heavily involves the triceps, and the upper back) and Smith machine upright row (which targets the shoulder muscles, mainly the deltoids and the trapezius muscles).

Varun reserves one full hour for cardio exercises on the third day. Running is great to have as a part of the cardio repertoire as it's not only a great way to get fitter but also improves mental well-being.

On the fourth day, the actor concentrates on building his back, triceps and abs. Some of the workouts done by him are barbell T-bar rows, barbell dead-lifts, seated cable rows, inverted rows, straight-arm pull-downs, one-arm dumb-bell rows, pull-downs and the bent-over barbell rows, among others, exclusively for his back. For his triceps, he works on seated overhead triceps extensions, skull crushers, the Smith machine close-grip bench presses and the standing overhead tricep extensions.

His basic gym routine for his abs is:

- 4×12 decline sit-ups
- 3×15 cable crunches
- 3×10/10 side dumb-bell bends
- 3×8 straight-leg sit-ups

For his lower abs, he does:

- 20 double crunches
- 30 Russian twists
- 20 hip raises
- 15/15 twisting lunges
- 20 sit-ups
- 20 double crunches
- 3 leg raises and hold

The fifth day is reserved for working on his legs. He does 15 reps and 5 sets of squats, followed by leg presses, leg extensions, leg curls and raise of calf muscles. He also focuses on his cardio workout.

On the sixth day, Varun opts for functional exercises to build up strength for action sequences and exercises throughout the day.

1. His session begins with air squats, which are full squats with no extra weight (barbell or dumb-bells).

2. He then shifts gear to overhead squats, holding a weight overhead.

3. After that, he moves on to front squats, in which a squat with barbell is racked in the front at shoulder level.

4. Next, he switches to jumping squats in which one jumps upwards after rising from each squat.

5. Then comes the skaters' samurai squats (also known as dumb-bell tricep extension with deep squat).

6. For the remaining part of the session, he does a plank up lat pull-over on a Swiss ball to target his abs, back and hips. It sculpts the core, chest, shoulders and back. These muscles are strengthened with pull-ups, pull-downs and rows.

7. Varun then moves on to do straight leg with squat thrusts, which are great exercises for total body conditioning.

8. Next on his schedule are hammer curls, lunges and presses which target the whole body.

9. Other than these, he does standing mountain climbers, shoulder presses with leg extension, good-morning presses (this exercise strengthens the core and increases flexibility), triceps kickback static lunges with lateral raise, bicycle crunches, dead-lifts with upright rows and clock push-ups that targets multiple muscles.

10. He also does close-grip triceps push-ups (which work the whole of the back upper arm), butt-kick woodchopper triceps dips (triceps kickbacks tone the triceps, the woodchopper exercise erases love handles and squats squeeze the butt), leg raise in reverse plank (targets the shoulders, legs and abs), side lunges with bicep curls (targets the inner and outer thighs, glutes, quads and biceps—a compound move that works the whole body and boosts the heart rate), the boat pose (strengthens the abs and deep hip flexor) and the triceps rope push-downs elbow extension. Finally, he does the ViPR circuit training (vitality, performance and reconditioning) for 10–20 minutes, which includes cardio exercises, to complete his day's routine.

Apart from all this, Varun also loves cycling and believes, 'It's the best way to get where you want.'[4]

Such an intense training regimen means he feels comfortable doing all his stunt scenes himself in his action movies.

One interesting fact about Varun's training schedule is that after every seven months, he takes a break and goes on a well-deserved fortnight-long 'holiday', where he abstains from all workouts. This is because he treats his body with care and does not want to push it to its limit. This helps expedite the body's recovery from fatigue and injuries.

Martial Arts

Varun is trained in viper martial arts. This Chinese martial-arts form, also known as snake boxing or fanged-snake style, imitates the movements of snakes. It is a style of Shaolin boxing made popular by Jackie Chan in the cult movie *Snake in the Eagle's Shadow* and later in *Five Deadly Venoms*. Proponents of this style claim that adopting the fluidity of snakes allows them to entwine with their opponents in defence and strike them from angles they wouldn't expect.

Varun, the Avid Dancer

An enthusiastic dancer, Varun believes that dancing is one of the best forms of aerobics. A vigorous dance routine helps burn a lot of calories and at the same time the body gains flexibility and agility. He loves dancing on a regular basis. In fact, his stellar physique and brilliant dance moves in *ABCD2 (Anybody Can Dance 2)*, released in 2015, won him a huge fan following worldwide. It was not easy for his co-star Shraddha Kapoor to match up to him.

Student of the Year

In *Student of the Year*, Varun had a scene where he had to come out of a swimming pool in barely-there briefs and for that he needed to have a chiselled body.

He worked out for an hour every day, combining a lot of cardio with weight training.

He also included yoga and TRX (total resistance exercise) in his regimen. TRX is an approach to resistance training that involves body-weight exercises by using a system of webbing ropes called suspension trainers. The exercises are done with the aim of improving mobility and joint stability, development of strength, balance and flexibility as well as to build up lean muscles, all the while using functional movements and dynamic positions.

Such exercises also helped Varun's dance routines and workouts.

To supplement his training regimen, Varun was put on a low-carb diet along with the basic supplements, ranging from protein to BCAA (branched-chain amino acids, which are especially helpful for maintaining muscle mass while on a calorie-deficit diet. They're particularly useful for bodybuilding competitors who take their physiques to the lean extreme). Varun got most of his protein intake from chicken, which he loves.

ABCD 2

In *ABCD 2*, Varun essayed the role of a professional dancer. Choreographer-turned-director Remo D'Souza, who made the film, asked Varun to sculpt a raw, lean body for the role of Suresh. This was communicated to his trainer, Sawant, who did extensive research on dancers and their fitness regimens. Most dancers, he found, had lean bodies without toned muscles. Many even sported six-pack abs without really concentrating much on achieving them.

As Sawant puts it: 'Their fitness was more functional than vanity-based. They have super-fit bodies with abs, and that was surprising. It's difficult to achieve that level of fitness, but the amount of dancing they did helped them easily burn every inch of unwanted fat.'[5]

Incidentally, Varun lost a total of 6 kg for the film, and Sawant was all praise for his dedication. He proudly declared Varun as one of his most dedicated disciples who would go to any length to achieve the desired look. All his hard work was evident in the film.

Varun would dance for long hours throughout the day and again work out both before and after the shoot. But Sawant faced another challenge. As Varun had to dance for longer hours towards the end of the movie, his muscle mass began to vanish. To counter that, Sawant kept his cardio to a bare minimum and upped his weight training to maintain muscle mass. Even his diet was changed. Initially, Varun had to maintain a low-carb, high-protein diet. But as shooting began, he was put on a high-carb and high-protein diet.

Prior to *ABCD2* in 2013, Varun had collaborated with Remo D'Souza to release a fitness DVD,

Pumpstart. This was a compilation of a dance routine that flexes thirteen major muscle groups in the body, choreographed by D'Souza.

Dishoom and *Badrinath Ki Dulhania*

Varun has not only maintained his well-sculpted frame over the years, but has taken the leap to train even harder whenever the scripts have demanded it. For *Dishoom*, he trained for three months without a break. He worked rigorously on a lean and mean look for a bare-bodied fight sequence in Sajid Nadiadwala's action drama, which also featured John Abraham and Jacqueline Fernandez.

He also increased his workout routine for *Badrinath Ki Dulhania* (sequel to *Humpty Sharma Ki Dulhania*). The twenty-nine-year-old *ABCD 2* actor changed his gym regimen to beef up for the role.

Judwaa 2

In September 2017, Varun appeared in a dual role as twins in his father David Dhawan's comedy sequel to Salman Khan starrer *Judwaa*. Varun put on and then shed weight for the double role in *Judwaa 2*, as one of the twins he portrays is lean and the other is buff. For the latter role, he had to show off his sculpted muscles, for which he trained hard under his trainer, Prashant Sawant.

Varun was on a high-protein, low-carb diet for the movie and had to eat every three hours. He was allowed to have carbohydrates only in the afternoon. Prashant said that while Varun looked muscular in *ABCD 2*, in *Judwaa 2*, he needed to go one step further. For that, he did a lot of martial arts and trained for one and a half hours daily for greater flexibility.

Varun's Diet Plan

Varun is as fastidious about his diet as he is about his daily exercise regimen. Of course, he allows himself his 'cheat days' to keep himself motivated, and can be seen on social media enjoying a slice of pizza, cheesecake, or even a chocolate milkshake. However, he is very particular about what he eats otherwise, and relishes healthy food and enjoys leading a physically fit lifestyle on the whole.

Breakfast

He begins his day with the most important meal—breakfast. Many tend to skip this exceptionally vital fare, hoping to shed some calories. However, they get it wrong, since skipping breakfast actually leads to a significant rise in calories, among other potentially toxic substances in the body, as recent research conducted by Johns Hopkins has revealed.[6]

'People skip breakfast thinking they're cutting calories, but by mid-morning and lunch, that person is starved,' says Milton Stokes, RD, MPH, chief dietitian for St. Barnabas Hospital in New York City. 'Breakfast skippers replace calories during the day with mindless nibbling, bingeing at lunch and dinner. They set themselves up for failure.'[7] Thus, most dietitians strongly stress on the importance of a healthy, nutritive breakfast.

Varun enjoys an omelette, oatmeal and a wholegrain wheat sandwich for breakfast. Then he hits the gym for a quick warm-up before heading off to shoots or appointments.

Lunch

Varun has a simple yet wholesome lunch, which consists of brown rice, broccoli and baked chicken. Broccoli offers high levels of immune system-boosting vitamin C, bone-strengthening vitamin K, and folate, which plays a strategic role in regulating cell growth and reproduction. It's also packed with glucosinolate compounds, such as sulforaphane and glucoraphanin, which help fight cancer.

Snacks

To battle sudden hunger pangs, Varun eats lotus seeds, which are a good source of protein, carbohydrates, fibre, magnesium, potassium, phosphorus, iron and zinc. High in fibre and low in calories, they enable weight loss. The low sodium and high magnesium content makes them beneficial for those suffering from heart diseases, high blood pressure, diabetes and obesity.

Varun also snacks on papayas (good for antioxidants, phytonutrients and flavonoids that prevent one's cells from undergoing free radical damage) and bananas, or else, skips solid food and opts for a protein shake.

Dinner

Varun ends the day with a meal of mixed greens and grilled fish. As is evident from his daily diet, Varun is extremely cautious about what he eats as he has a family history of diabetes and obesity. (A balanced diet with minimal sugar and carbs is important for those who have a family history of diabetes.)

Varun Dhawan is not just another young Bollywood star who found success thanks to his famous father. He has worked hard and practised discipline and restraint to prove his success. His daily routine of rigorous exercise and his well-charted diet plans have proved beyond doubt that Varun is a man who can go to any length to prove his worth. He has stretched himself and his goals with utter sincerity and his strict lifestyle is an inspiration for all youngsters.

5

Farhan Akhtar: Body and Brains

Bollywood Background

Farhan is not just an actor. Or a director. Or a singer. Or a screenwriter. The list could go on. He's a multitalented, multifaceted prime product of Bollywood. Born in Mumbai to screenwriter Javed Akhtar and actor Honey Irani, Farhan is one of two children. His sibling Zoya Akhtar is another talented director who made her mark with *Zindagi Na Milegi Dobara*.

Farhan made a splash in Bollywood with his directorial debut *Dil Chahta Hai,* which received immense critical acclaim. It was a path-breaking film, portraying the life of contemporary urban young men, depicting their hopes, dreams, love, friendships, and transformations in a very nuanced manner. The film resonated with people of all ages, especially the youth. Over the years, the film has attained a cult status and become a classic.

After winning a National Award for *Dil Chahta Hai*, Farhan went on to make *Lakshya* (2004), the highly successful *Don* (2006) and *Don 2* (2011). He won a second National Award for best feature film as producer for *Rock On!!* in 2008, making his official debut as an actor in this film.

He went on to act in, produce and write dialogues for the very successful and acclaimed *Zindagi Na Milegi Dobara* (2011), which was directed by his sister, Zoya. This film won him two Filmfare awards, including one for best supporting actor. In the same year, Farhan directed *Don 2*, his most successful commercial venture till date. Then in 2013, he portrayed Milkha Singh in the film *Bhaag Milkha Bhaag*, which not only earned him the Filmfare Award for best actor but also required the most significant transformation physically.

Fitness Fanatic

Samir Jauhar, Farhan's personal trainer since 2004, reveals how passionate Farhan is about fitness: 'It's not just a hobby for him. It's his lifestyle.' Farhan is highly motivated and loves working out. But just to avoid boredom and break the monotony, Samir keeps changing his workouts. 'He is a perfectionist. I'm a perfectionist. So this is what happens when two perfectionists meet. They never compromise. They are true to themselves.' Samir calls Farhan his best student. He follows instructions to the T and always does what he's told. He's very particular about his workout routines. 'I'm so proud of him because at the age of forty-one he managed to achieve a physique that required an intense transformation for his role in *Bhaag Milkha Bhaag*. How many forty-one-year-olds can do that?'

Samir mentions that Farhan's body is ectomorphic or lean. If he doesn't work out, he loses weight instead of gaining it. Ectomorph body types have a linear physique and are fragile or delicately built. They find it difficult to gain weight or add muscle. They are slim boned, long-limbed and lithe. This body type is most common among models. Male ectomorphs struggle to increase their muscle mass as they tend to look very lean and thin. At the same time, as they grow older, their super-fast metabolism slows down and they start gaining weight. But this is when male ectomorphs have an opportunity to turn this body fat into muscle. Farhan is a highly committed and focused ectomorph body type. Samir greatly admires Farhan's persistence and fitness goals.

Sports Enthusiast

Farhan is a volleyball enthusiast and manages to take time out to play the game at least once or twice a week. He's also passionate about skydiving. Samir mentions that Farhan has recently been going to Spain every year, where he takes a break from work. There he makes it a point to go skydiving. So, even on holidays Farhan manages to keep things action-packed as he's naturally energetic and athletic. Recently, Farhan has also taken to cycling. On holidays abroad, he hires a cycle to travel around, and also goes to the beach wherever possible for a swim. In fact, after he's back from a holiday, Samir has no trouble getting him in shape as Farhan manages to stay quite fit.

Being physically active throughout the year helps Farhan always keep his fitness levels at a peak. It also means he does not have to diet or change his eating habits drastically in order to lose weight.

Farhan's Day-to-day Fitness Tips

- Regular routine: Farhan is very particular about sticking to a fitness routine. He works out every day for two and a half hours. This includes a forty-five-minute ab workout, followed by a trainer routine that changes every week.

He also plays volleyball and swims at least two to three times a week. This keeps his body flexible and agile. He rests on Sundays or plays some sport.

- Finding a balance: Farhan finds ways to keep stress at bay. Exercising is a great stress-buster, so it is important to find ways to balance out your work and leisure activities that help you keep fit. Farhan finds exercise to be a fantastic way to release stress and thus maintain emotional balance.
- Time management: Despite his busy schedule, Farhan finds time to do the things he loves, and stresses on the importance of inculcating these physical activities in one's life. If you have a favourite sport, then find time for it. His way of ensuring he keeps active apart from going to the gym is by taking time out to swim, play football and volleyball, all activities he really enjoys. So, ensuring you have a stable and regular exercise regimen throughout the year should be your aim.
- Beating genetic factors: One does not put on weight only because of ones genes. You must do whatever it takes to keep fit and maintain your weight.
- Avoid alcohol: If you can, try to avoid alcohol. Or drink a limited amount occasionally if it is an integral part of your lifestyle.
- Avoid fried foods: Avoid fatty, deep-fried and junk foods. Farhan avoids carbs as well and has eliminated rotis from his diet completely.

- Cycle at least once a week to avoid the legs becoming stiff between workouts.
- Run up the stairs to build your stamina.

Foodie or Health Nut

Farhan likes the occasional ice cream (only one scoop!) after dinner or a piece or two of dark chocolate. He has no other food cravings or indulgences. 'Actually he's very focused and eating healthy has become a way of life for him,' says Samir about his favourite trainee celeb. Farhan has trained his mind and body to such a degree that he eats clean and healthy throughout the year.

So trying to eat healthy just before a shoot is not his eating pattern. He just makes minor adjustments in his diet while preparing for a role. On a regular day, Farhan eats about 150 g of meat in a meal, but on pre-shoot days, he restricts it between 75 and 100 g. Before a shoot, he also cuts down or avoids oil, salt and spices but otherwise enjoys his salads with healthy dressings. Farhan eats a lot of salads, grilled or sautéed in olive oil, with fish, turkey or chicken. His diet also includes a lot of quinoa, couscous, buckwheat pasta, and brown, red and black rice. He prefers having fruits like berries (strawberries, blueberries, blackberries and others), oranges and watermelon. He does have the occasional banana, but in a protein smoothie. Being very conscious of the portions is another habit that helps him stay in shape.

Farhan strongly believes that it is very important that one gets used to a healthy and nutritious way of eating, as it is not something to be adopted occasionally. It should become a part of your lifestyle. Alcohol is one of the aspects to which he applies this rule quite strictly. He rarely drinks and even if he does, it's usually a pint of beer on social occasions or holidays. He also totally abstains from smoking.

At parties, he generally avoids eating the food that is being served and instead prefers home-cooked food meticulously prepared by his chef. He does not have any inclinations for restaurant food either.

Diet Chart for Regular Days

- **Breakfast:** 6 egg whites + 1 slice multigrain bread + 1 glass of orange/carrot/vegetable juice.
                        Or
  1 bowl of muesli with yoghurt and juice + 1 avocado.
- **Mid-morning snack:** 1 protein shake (whey protein isolate).
- **Lunch:** 100–150 g of chicken/turkey/fish, lots of salad with dressing, a bowl of yellow dal (he is fond of eating dal), 2 multigrain rotis/a bowl of brown/red/black rice.

- **Evening snack:** 1 bowl of nuts/moong salad/ chickpea salad and fruit/fruit smoothie with protein supplement.
- **Dinner:** Grilled chicken/fish/turkey, salad with lots of vegetables (broccoli, beans, asparagus, etc.). He avoids rice at night.

The *Bhaag Milkha Bhaag* Transformation

Endurance Is the Name of the Game

Farhan's most noticeable body transformation so far has been for his film *Bhaag Milkha Bhaag*, wherein Farhan played the 'Flying Sikh,' the name by which Milkha Singh came to be known. Milkha Singh was the only Indian athlete to win an individual gold medal at the Commonwealth Games until Krishna Poona in 2010. Milkha has also won gold medals in the 1958 and 1962 Asian Games. He was awarded the Padma Shri in honour of his sporting achievements.

Samir reveals that when director Rakeysh Omprakash Mehra gave him the script to work on Farhan's look, 'his reference point was Brad Pitt in the movie *Fight Club*.' He had to achieve that look for Farhan.

The training sessions began in November 2011. For the next thirteen months, Farhan toiled, sweated and sweated some more. He finished training for the film in December 2012.

Farhan trained with Samir as well as the professional athletic coach Melwyn Crasto.

The athletic training sessions were conducted under the supervision and guidance of Coach Melvyn in Mumbai's Priyadarshini Park, which has a synthetic track on which Farhan had to practise running with spikes, like a trained athlete. The training sessions were designed to increase Farhan's flexibility and enable him to sprint like a professional athlete.

Farhan would begin training at 6.30 a.m. and do ninety minutes of sprints and flexibility exercises. Because running has a neuromuscular component, he was taught drills that broke the monotony of running and helped coordinate body movements. These drills, referred to as the ABC of running, are essentially isolated phases of the gait cycle—the knee lift, upper leg motion and push. These exercises helped Farhan become a near professional runner.

The three looks in the film (which are all vastly different physique-wise) that Farhan sported were developed in reverse order—the film was shot from end to beginning. His last and most muscular look was achieved first. Initially, Farhan weighed around 66 kg, which was slowly beefed up to 75 kg to achieve the muscular and ripped body audiences across the country saw. Next he dropped 15 kg for the part in which he joined the army, which took three and a half months. They had to be careful to do this by reducing the muscle definition.

The exercise routine for Farhan was flawlessly planned and executed by Samir. The primary focus was to make him look athletic and add muscle or bulk to his ectomorph body type. Samir would change his workouts every fifteen days so that his body would not get used to a particular kind of workout. For the first six months, apart from strength training, Samir also introduced hypertrophy strength training (HST) whereby the muscles thicken and induce the fastest growth over an extended period without the use of steroids. It involves increasing the load on muscles consistently with every session. This increases activity within a muscle cell and makes it more sensitive to incoming nutrients for repair.

Farhan also trained with heavy weights and followed the Tabata principle, which places emphasis on training for short fixed bursts. All this along with endurance training gave Farhan the impetus needed to achieve the look.

For the first month and a half, Farhan trained for one and a half hours, twice a day. In the mornings he trained with coach Melwyn to increase his flexibility, in the evenings he concentrated on weight training. After six weeks, Samir increased Farhan's workouts to thrice a day. So it became one hour of running in the morning, one hour of functional training, involving core workouts and stretching in the afternoon, and one and a half hours of strength training in the evening. After these intense sessions Farhan had to be in bed by 10.30 p.m. latest. It was very necessary that his body got enough rest and recuperation to heal or build up muscle tissue.

Farhan followed this rigorous routine for almost one and a half years. He also adapted extremely well to this austere lifestyle and gave it his 100 per cent. Samir is full of admiration for the actor, especially how he managed this at the age of forty-one.

Bhaag Milkha Bhaag was initially shot in Nubra Valley, Ladakh. Farhan and his training team reached fifteen days before the shooting began. Samir reveals, 'It was a dessert with no connectivity. But Farhan made use of the terrain and cycled a lot on mountain trails.'

The dietary requirements expected to be followed by the actor were no less gruelling. All his food was carefully weighed out before being prepared and served, to monitor how many grams of proteins, carbs and fats he was ingesting. However, he was given well-balanced meals to suit his body's requirements.

Salt in his diet was practically non-existent, or as Sameer says, 'Naam ke vaaste.' A low-sodium diet ensured that he didn't have water retention issues. He was allowed only two teaspoons of olive oil in a day, and rice and bread were completely eliminated from his diet. His only cheat food was a big glass of lassi every fifteen days.

For his muscular look, Farhan's calorie intake was about 3500 in a day, which was reduced to 1800 calories a day for his leaner look.

Then there were two phases in the film, Samir reveals, for which Farhan was put solely on a liquid diet for five days. 'There is a skipping scene in the movie which depicts this physique transition from lean to bulky.' His liquid diet consisted of coconut water, plain water, fruit juices, fruit shakes and green tea.

Samir reveals that Rakeysh Mehra brought in trained athletes from universities all over the world to shoot for the running scenes. And these athletes thought that Farhan was an athlete too and not an actor! It just goes to show the kind of effort put in by Farhan to achieve this effect was phenomenal. His athletic prowess is no doubt evident in the film. That he bagged numerous awards, even internationally, confirms this unequivocally.

The Workout Drill

This workout routine was incorporated into the thirteen-month programme that Farhan followed. This was a part of the basic routine at the start of the training for the film. Afterwards, his workouts became far more intensive and rigorous. Samir played it by ear and kept modifying and adjusting according to the director's requirements. However, these workouts will go a long way in keeping any person fit and also help them achieve a fabulous body.

Weeks 1 and 2

Day 1
Chest and Triceps
- Flat bench-presses: 15 reps (4 sets)
- Dumb-bell incline presses: 15 reps (4 sets)
- Incline flyes: 15 reps (4 sets)
- Dips on machine: 15 reps (4 sets)
- Tricep push-downs: 15 reps (4 sets)
- Skull crushers: 15 reps (4 sets)

Day 2
- Running: 40 minutes

Day 3
Legs, Shoulders and Abs
- Squats: 15 reps (5 sets)
- Leg extensions: 15 reps (5 sets)
- Leg curls: 15 reps (5 sets)
- Calf-raises: 15 reps (5 sets)
- Seated military-presses: 12 reps (4 sets)

- Lateral raises: 12 reps (4 sets)
- Front raises: 12 reps (4 sets)
- Cable crunches: 100 reps (5 sets)

Day 4
- Swimming: 40 minutes

Day 5
Back and Biceps
- Cable front pull-downs: 15 reps (5 sets)
- Seated back-rows: 15 reps (5 sets)
- Standing alternative dumb-bell curls: 15 reps (5 sets)
- Concentration curls: 15 reps (5 sets)

Day 6
- Cross trainer: 60 minutes

Day 7
- Rest

Weeks 3 and 4

Day 1
Chest and Back
- Flat bench-presses: 15 reps (5 sets)
- Dumb-bell incline presses: 15 reps (5 sets)
- One-arm dumb-bell rows: 15 reps (5 sets)
- Seated back-rows: 15 reps (5 sets)

- Shrugs: 15 reps (5 sets)

Day 2
- Running: 40 minutes

Day 3
Legs, Shoulders and Abs
- Squats: 15 reps (5 sets)
- Stiff-leg dead-lifts: 15 reps (5 sets)
- Calf raises: 15 reps (5 sets)

Day 4
- Swimming: 50 minutes

Day 5
Arms
- Dumb-bell curls: 12 reps (4 sets)
- Straight-bar curls: 12 reps (4 sets)
- Close-grip bench presses: 12 reps (4 sets)
- Tricep push-downs: 12 reps (4 sets)

Day 6
- Cross trainer: 60 minutes

Weeks 5 to 8

- This workout was performed 5 days a week
- Seated rows + incline flyes (superset): 15 reps (5 sets)

- Leg extensions + front raises (superset): 15 reps (5 sets)
- Cable curls + tricep push-downs (superset): 15 reps (5 sets)
- Side bends: 100 reps (5 sets)
- Crunches: 100 reps (5 sets)
- Leg raises: 100 reps (5 sets)
- Running: 50 minutes
- Rest for 30 seconds between every set. After finishing 5 sets, rest for 3 minutes and start the next superset.

Weeks 9 to 12

- This workout was performed 6 days a week
- T-bar rows + cable crossovers (superset): 15 reps (8 sets)
- Leg extensions + front presses with dumb-bells (superset): 15 reps (8 sets)
- Preacher curls + push-downs with rope (superset): 15 reps (8 sets)
- Side bends: 200 reps (5 sets)
- Crunches: 200 reps (5 sets)
- Leg raises: 200 reps (5 sets)
- Running: 50 minutes
- Rest for 30 seconds and move to the next set. After finishing 5 sets, rest for 3 minutes and start the next superset.

Focus on Particular Body Parts

Shoulders

Lateral raises helped him develop rounded and muscled shoulders. Along with that, he did 15 sets of front raises with dumb-bells regularly.

Abs

For his eight-pack, Farhan did around 2500–3000 crunches, leg raises, side bends and other abdominal exercises daily.

Legs

300 counts of squats, jump squats, lunges, leg presses and extensions and 100 calf-raises gave Farhan the runner's legs.

Biceps

He got his bulging biceps by doing 12 sets of exercises such as curls, preacher curls, cable workouts and concentration curls regularly.

The *Wazir* Look

For *Wazir*, Farhan wanted the look of a tough cop. In fact, says Samir, Farhan looked more ripped in this film than he did in *Bhaag Milkha Bhaag*. But the training period was of a much shorter duration.

Farhan trained intensively for five weeks. Samir focused mainly on strength training with heavy weights but a lower number of reps to bulk up his muscles.

Farhan trained for about two hours six times a week in a routine called split training. This is a form of training in which specific muscle groups are trained on specific days of the week or at predetermined intervals. This is opposed to training the entire body with each workout. There are a multitude of possible combinations one could use when designing this type of programme.

Split training is used to bulk up muscles within a short period of time. Samir focused on training one small and one large muscle on a particular day. Small muscles include the triceps and biceps while large muscles include the back legs and chest. For a small muscle he would not do more than 12 sets and for large muscles it was not more than 16 sets. So although the number of sets were less, the weights used were heavy.

Ab exercises were done every day but broken into segments. So starting on Mondays, he would focus on exercising the obliques or side muscles of the abdomen. Then on Tuesday he worked on the upper abs and on Wednesday on the lower abdominal muscles. The whole cycle was repeated Thursday onwards. So, in essence, he was training the same muscle twice a week.

The routine he followed was:

- Monday: Chest and biceps with abs
- Tuesday: Legs and shoulders with abs
- Wednesday: Back and triceps with abs
- Thursday: Chest and biceps with abs
- Friday: Legs and shoulders with abs
- Saturday: Back and triceps with abs

His diet consisted of complex carbs and proteins in every meal; he ate five to six times in a day. This diet was unlike the one he followed for *Bhaag Milkha Bhaag,* where carbs were eliminated from his diet completely. His main sources of protein were chicken, fish, turkey and protein powders. He also drank 4 litres of water every day.

The 'Supermodel' Look Workout

In March 2017, Samir got a call from Farhan, saying he needed to look like a supermodel for a magazine photo-shoot, and that too in eight weeks. He wanted to know if Samir could plan out a workout accordingly.

Samir being the achiever he is, didn't back down from the challenge. It is no wonder then, that Farhan has such faith in him and surrenders to the trainer's expertise completely. Needless to say, the duo achieved its goal within the stipulated time frame. Samir says, 'This workout put him in the best shape of his life. He was beefier and more muscular.'

Of course, Farhan trained very hard to achieve this look. When actors sign up for a film, filmmakers lay down certain conditions. The actors give it their all and this is perhaps the reason for their superlative success.

To get in shape, Farhan would wake up at 5.30 a.m. every day. Then Samir and the actor would hit the streets of Mumbai, sometimes cycling as far as Nariman Point or the Gateway of India all the way from Bandra and then back. The goal was to do 22–30 km every day, for eight weeks.

After finishing his cycling circuit, Farhan would have a quick glass of orange/carrot juice and then hit the gym for a two-hour workout with Samir.

As he regularly plays volleyball, he continued doing that rigorously twice a week. This added that extra zing to his already intense workout schedule.

Samir put Farhan on strength and functional training schedules because Farhan has a high metabolism rate and tends to lose weight when he's on a high-powered workout regimen.

Samir also monitored Farhan's water intake. Samir is of the opinion that it's not advisable to drink more than 5 litres of water in a day. Excess consumption just flushes out the essential minerals and vitamins stored in the body.

During this time, Farhan would have six egg whites for breakfast along with watered dahi. He was also on a no-carb diet, which meant no roti, bread or even rice. He added salmon and lots of salad to achieve that lean look. Salmon is a great source of protein and also aids weight control. It has few calories but at the same time is rich in omega-3 fatty acids, which may help in weight loss and soothe stiff joints.

Conclusion

Over the last few years, Farhan has managed to up the level of fitness in the industry due to his dedication and willingness to change his look for a role. And a part of the credit goes to his trainer.

Samir has been his one and only trainer since 2001. Samir reveals that the actor takes his work very seriously and gets into minor details about the training and diet routine he has to follow for any film. He's very meticulous. Samir says, 'I'm very comfortable working with him as we share a very long relationship.'

Samir has trained many celebrities. But his admiration for Farhan remains undiminished. His perfectionism, unwavering focus and uncompromising discipline always sets him apart. But from a man of so many talents, we expect nothing less.

6

Tiger Shroff: The Sculpted Dancer

Does the name Jai Hemant Shroff sound familiar? No? Take a guess. Still at a loss? Well, he is the man everyone swooned over as he danced to the beats of 'Beparwah', the climactic song from his recent movie *Munna Michael*. He's none other than Tiger Shroff, son of ex-Bollywood hunk, Jackie Shroff, the man who took Bollywood by storm in the 1980s with his husky voice and good looks. Jai Hemant, or Tiger, as everyone calls him, is his son and the man who raised the bar of fitness to a new level in Bollywood. Though shy and reluctant to talk about it, it is no more a secret in the industry that Aamir Khan took this debutant's help in rebuilding his physique for *Dhoom 3*.

Despite a very down-to-earth upbringing, away from the spotlight, Tiger has been a fitness and dance pro since his childhood days. He and his sister, Krishna, three years his junior, attended the American School of Bombay with Shraddha Kapoor and Athiya Shetty. Shraddha Kapoor in an interview once mentioned she was a big fan of Tiger since schooldays, and that he was a great sportsman. 'I often watched him play basketball like a pro,' she said.

Tiger has been popular among his friends and contemporaries since his schooldays. Martial arts have always been his forte. For him, martial arts are not just for building muscles and staying fit, they are synonymous with meditation and intense focus on something, like an ancient samurai on the battlefield. This lithe actor started taking lessons in different forms of martial arts since the age of four and still continues to learn new forms and moves.

Standing tall at 5 feet 11 inches, Tiger has inherited his parents' good looks and a lean and athletic physique. He has always been a sports freak, and there was a time when he thought of playing football professionally and was a part of the soccer circuit. However, before long, he realized that football is not considered a major game in India and does not hold much promise for the future at the time. So, he decided to channel his talents to other fields.

One of the best dancers among the many new Bollywood entrants in recent times, Tiger Shroff has an extremely fluid body, and it is sheer pleasure watching him dance. His talent has been skilfully put to the fore by Sabbir Khan in his movie *Munna Michael*. The essence and spirit of the film is captured by a dashing Tiger, moving stealthily like a serpent. For the 'Beparwah' song sequence, he was specially trained by a team of domestic and international choreographers who had earlier helped with projects involving global performers, such as the late Michael Jackson, Janet Jackson and Jennifer Lopez. If you have watched *Step Up* and the new *Ghostbusters*, you will know what a great team Tiger was with. The experienced team was left spellbound by Tiger's fitness, skill and performance.

Even Hrithik Roshan has publicly hailed the youngster as the next dance sensation to hit Bollywood.[1] But all this fame has not affected Tiger. He continues to be a fitness freak whose workout routine remains unchanged despite his commitments and busy schedule, mostly because his time management is excellent.

Tiger had been receiving movie offers from Bollywood bigwigs for quite some time before he made his debut, but he refused many because he believed his father's towering presence in Bollywood would overshadow his efforts. It required a lot of persuasion and assurance from others before he mustered enough courage to give acting a shot. Finally, he took the plunge when director Sabbir

Khan offered him the lead role in his romantic thriller *Heropanti*. The movie catapulted Tiger into the big league instantly. Though there were mixed reviews about the movie as a whole, veteran film critics like Subhash Jha and Taran Adarsh were all praise for Tiger's acting prowess and the action scenes. His portrayal also won him a nomination for the Filmfare Award for the best male debut that year. Tiger bagged his first best debutant hero award at Stardust Awards for *Heropanti* and his first magazine cover was also with the same publication. For the cover shoot with ace photographer Gaurav Sethi, Tiger Shroff came with basic fitness equipment and would do his crunches and stretches on the set for a perfect chiselled look. His bare-bodied cover shoot became a bestseller and the making of the video went viral.

Tiger is a health freak and hits the gym daily without a break. He is extremely particular about his workout regimen and daily food intake. He and his mate Suraj Pancholi are often spotted hanging out together at the gym where they both train. Tiger is still very fond of playing football and practises dribbling regularly on the field. He is also into gymnastics and practises it to keep his body supple and flexible.

With his debut film receiving appreciation from Bollywood veterans, Tiger felt encouraged to focus more on his fitness and continued his tremendous hard work. His well-toned athletic, muscular body is the result of sheer tenacity, a balanced diet, proper supplementation and adequate rest. A diehard Bruce Lee fan, Tiger has made sure martial-arts training and kick-boxing are a significant part of his regular regimen. The Hong Kong and American actor, martial-arts icon and film director Bruce Lee has had such an influence on Tiger that when he was asked which biopic would be his dream movie, Tiger promptly replied he would love to portray Bruce Lee or Michael Jackson. In his words to *Stardust*: 'While I grew up watching Lee's martial-arts sequences in films, and I have worshipped Jackson ever since I can remember.'

Among all kinds of martial arts, Tiger loves kick-boxing as it not only helps in sculpting muscles, but is also a stress buster. Kick-boxing moves can burn up to 500 calories an hour, and targets abs, shoulders, thighs and butt, all in just one workout. It helps get over the boredom of sweating it out at the gym doing the same exercises every day.

Tiger is already a practitioner of taekwondo (karate and Korean martial-arts combined) and wushu (a traditional Chinese martial-arts form that amalgamates all kinds of moves) and they form an integral part of his daily routine. Not only does Tiger work on these arts on his own, but he has also trained under professionals. He has coached under national-level gymnast Ziley Mawai, and together they have worked on extremely tough, gravity-defying stunts like wall-flips and high-octane jumps. Such stunts are dangerous as one wrong foot placement can lead to a ligament or even a muscle tear. Tiger's toned body and fearless spirit has always helped him perform such stunts without any help or someone to stand in for him.

Tiger Shroff's Workout Routine for *Heropanti*

Tiger Shroff's menacing action hero look in *Heropanti* added to the stunt sequences, which he did without using a body double. His aerial moves with kicks were highly appreciated. In a *Stardust* interview, he talked about some of these stunts, particularly citing one, 'There was a scene where I had to do three backflips continuously and pick up my jacket the third time. That required perfect timing and was extremely difficult.'

In fact, stunt specialists have not stopped praising Tiger's daring parkour sequence, which lasted for six minutes and thirty seconds, the longest in Indian cinema so far. Parkour is a training discipline that was developed in France by Raymond Belle, later built on by his son David. The movements are developed from military obstacle course training and include simple to complex exercise forms like running, climbing, swinging, vaulting, jumping, rolling and quadrupedal movement.

Tiger wished to take up this extreme and challenging art form before *Heropanti* as parkour-sequence movements are most suitable for getting from one point to another in a complex environment, without assistive equipment. It also happens to be the fastest and most efficient way of keeping fit. Tiger spent three months training rigorously in order to perfect the tough, challenging sequences required for the film. According to reports, multiple cameras were used for the shot to capture every nuance in its entirety.

Tiger's Weekly Workout

Tiger maintains a strict workout regimen and works out all seven days of the week, focusing on different parts of the body.

Monday:
- The week begins with back exercises that include a set of 12 pull-ups and dips (4–8 reps). Pull-ups develop the brachialis and brachio-radialis muscles of the arms. So, all those who would love to flaunt muscular arms, do not miss these exercises. Located near the elbow, these muscles

help move the forearm, biceps and shoulder joints.

- Tiger rounds off the pull-ups and dips with 4 sets of lateral machine pull-downs (80–85 kg) of (4–8 reps). The pull-down exercise is a strength-training exercise designed to develop the latissimus dorsi muscle. Then he moves on to a cable lat pull-down where the handle is moved via a cable pulley. The standard pull-down motion is a compound movement that requires dynamic muscle work.

- Next he does 12 sets of low one-arm dumb-bell rolls of 100 kg (4–8 reps). This helps increase and widen the back, while requires two types of movements: One is a pulling movement from overhead downward, while the other is where one pulls against resistance from a position in front of the body into the torso. Dumb-bells aid long-range motion and help to concentrate on each side of the back while exercising. Dumb-bell rolls assist the movement of the fan-shaped latissiumus dorsi muscles running from underneath the arms down to the lower back of the body.

Tuesday:

- Tiger lays a lot of stress on building muscle mass and strength around the chest. To do this, he begins with 12 sets of flat barbell bench-presses

(4–8 reps). The primary muscles that are worked in a bench press are the triceps and pecs.

- This is followed by 12 sets of incline bench-presses (4–8 reps). The incline bench activates and develops the upper chest muscles.
- Tiger then switches to 12 sets of dumb-bell presses (4–8 reps). The dumb-bell chest press is similar to the bench press and works on the chest muscles, shoulders, and triceps.
- He rounds off the day's regimen with 12 sets of chest flyes (4–8 reps). The chest fly or pectoral fly (or pec fly) primarily works the pectoralis major muscles to move the arms horizontally forward.

Wednesday:
- Wednesday is legs day for Tiger and begins with 4 sets of squats (4–8 reps) with 190-kg weight on the shoulders. Squats not only help build the leg muscles (including quadriceps, hamstrings and calves), but also work practically every single muscle of the body, helping to improve both upper- and lower-body strength.
- Tiger then strengthens the hamstrings by switching to 4 sets of hamstring curls (4–8 reps) with 90-kg weight.
- He does step-ups to strengthen the legs, and improve stability and balance.

- Next, his strength is tested as he lifts 4 sets of barbells (4–8 reps).
- He rounds off the day's exercise with 4 sets of free squats (4–8 reps).

Thursday:
- Tiger makes sure to reserve Thursdays for arms. He begins the day with 12 sets of Olympic barbell curls with 60-kg weight (4–8 reps). The classic Olympic bar bicep-curl builds bicep strength.
- This is followed with 12 sets of dumb-bell curls with 32-kg weights (4–8 reps).
- He then switches to 12 sets of reverse curls with 30-kg weight (4–8 reps). Reverse curl develops strength for a better grip. Developing this area helps lift heavier stuff for a longer period of time.
- The next 12 sets of close-grip barbell presses (4–8 reps) help develop the triceps.
- Tiger's next item is 12 sets of press-downs (4–8 reps). A push-down is a strength-training exercise used for strengthening the triceps muscles in the back of the arm.
- The exercise is completed by pushing an object downward against resistance. His exercise regimen ends after completing 12 sets of skull crushers with 68-kg weight (4–8 reps). Skull crushers that stimulate the entire triceps muscle group in the upper arm.

Friday:

- Tiger has Fridays slotted for shoulder exercises and begins with 12 sets of knee and shoulder presses with 90-kg weight (4–8 reps). This exercise strengthens the upper body.
- The 12 sets of military presses (4–8 reps) help him build a strong and muscular upper body, pushing his broad sculpted shoulders to their limits.
- He then switches to doing 6 sets of lateral raises (4–8 reps) using dumb-bells, to strengthen the entire shoulder, with emphasis on the sides of the deltoid muscles.
- This is followed by 6 sets of lateral raises (4–8 reps). The exercise helps ensure smooth motion and a fluid body.
- Tiger ends the day's workout with 12 sets of rear flyes with 40-kg weight (4–8 reps). Reverse-fly exercises with weight target the muscles in the upper back and work in the rhomboid muscles of the upper-back and shoulder region.

Saturday:

- Unlike Aamir Khan, Tiger doesn't rest his muscles on Saturdays and Sundays. Saturday begins with weight training exercise.
- Tiger starts off with 12 sets of squats with 100-kg weight (4–8 reps).

- He progresses to 12 sets of kneel and press with 50-kg weight (4–8 reps).
- He ends the day's workout with 12 sets of jumping push-ups (4–8 reps). This exercise not only increases speed and strength, but also skills via motor control as the body loses points of contact in the hands as they go off the ground.

Sunday:
- Tiger schedules his ab exercises for Sunday and begins with 12 sets of crunches (12 reps). The crunch is one of the most common abdominal exercises that primarily works the rectus abdominis muscle and the obliques.
- He turns to doing 12 sets of hanging reverse crunches (10–12 reps). Hanging reverse crunches are an excellent exercise to build lower abdominals. Then he goes for 12 sets of 10-kg weight-loaded reverse crunches (10–12 reps). The reverse crunch strengthens the abdominal muscles while placing less strain on the back and neck than a regular crunch. This exercise helps Tiger get and maintain those perfect six-pack abs.

His regimen is completed after doing 12 sets of standing and seated calf-presses (10–12 reps). Standing raises target the gastrocnemius, the ball-shaped muscle on the inside of the leg. This is what people traditionally think of, when picturing the calf muscle. Seated raises target the soleus, a longer muscle running underneath the gastrocnemius and on the outside of the lower leg.

Tiger Shroff's dedication and strict exercise regimen has helped him earn many laurels. In July 2014, shortly after the success of *Heropanti*, Kukkiwon (World Taekwondo Headquarters) bestowed him with an honorary taekwondo 5th-degree black belt. In the World Taekwondo Federation, students holding 1st–3rd dan (grade) are considered instructors, but generally have much to learn. Students who hold a 4th–6th dan are considered masters and must be at least eighteen years old. Those who hold a 7th–9th dan are considered grand masters. To be a grand master, the age requirement is to be at least forty and above. This prestigious award came his way when Kukkiwon officials watched him executing jaw-dropping, gravity-defying action scenes and complex yet beautifully synchronized martial-arts sequences, and were highly impressed.

Tiger's martial-arts skills were probably recognized because he was considered the right candidate—an ideal youth icon, who can inspire youngsters and the vulnerable to take up martial arts and self-defence training in order to protect themselves. This was indeed a rare honour for the actor, as he had never taken training from any taekwondo institute, but perfected the martial art to such a degree that the institute honoured him for his feat.

Tiger is not just disciplined about working out but also about this diet. These tips are great for non-vegetarians to adopt. However, if you have an underlying condition, please consult your doctor before incorporating these into your daily diet. Do remember that Tiger eats these according to how much he works out. If your workout routine is less intensive, adjust accordingly.

- Tiger's diet contains plenty of non-vegetarian protein and dietary fibre. These are essential for developing and maintaining muscle, so make sure to include these in your diet if you are trying to gain muscle tone.
- The day should always start with a healthy and proper breakfast—the very first and most important meal of the day after starving overnight for eight to nine hours. These days one sees teenagers skipping breakfast and crash-dieting. This is dangerous and should be avoided.
- A nutrient-fortified breakfast helps rejuvenate the body and mind, prevents muscle breakdown and provides energy for the rest of the day. Tiger has an early breakfast that consists of

eight egg whites and oatmeal. Egg white has several benefits and is an amazing source of protein without a lot of calories. This helps build muscles without adding on cholesterol and body fat. Oatmeal is a whole grain that adds fibre and nutrients to our body. It is also a rich source of iron, magnesium and vitamin B, and is considered a superfood. That provides the much-needed energy Tiger requires to follow the day's hectic schedule.

- Mid-morning before lunch, Tiger snacks on a glassful of power-boosting whey shake and dry fruits and nuts. Dried fruits like apricots, raisins, prunes and figs contain high amounts of beta carotene, vitamin E, iron, magnesium, potassium, niacin and calcium. Nuts like almonds, cashew nuts, pistachios, walnuts and dates are all packed with omega-3 fatty acids, protein, copper, calcium, potassium, etc., and boost energy levels.

- Tiger sticks to brown rice with boiled chicken and vegetables for lunch.

- His evening snack includes a protein shake. This is followed by a rigorous gymnastics session.

- A good night's sleep rejuvenates the body, and Tiger hits the bed early after his frugal dinner of boiled or lightly sautéed fish and broccoli.

- He abstains from fatty and oily food and drinks plenty of water to detoxify his system.

For Tiger, a good night's sleep is a must and hence he usually avoids any kind of late-night parties. 'Early to bed and early to rise is the mantra for success in life,' he says. Sound sleep is vital for a toned physique, so one should never compromise on one's sleep schedule. 'Leave all your worries for tomorrow and go for uninterrupted sleep. Your damaged cells will be replaced or rejuvenated, your system will work harmoniously and you will feel refreshed and ready to move on after a good night's sleep.'

Some Tips from Tiger Shroff to Keep Fit

- Eat healthy, stay healthy. Give up addictions, like hard drinks and smoking.
- If you are joining a gym, always go to a well-known or familiar gym and start working under the guidance of a trainer. Wrong exercises can harm your body for a lifetime; even overdoing it is not advisable.

Tiger's sincerity as well as perseverance have paid off well. Following his debut, a string of offers came his way and *Baaghi* and *A Flying Jatt* were both released in 2016. Though the films did not perform too well at the box office, his work was lauded by all and inspired both professionals and amateurs alike to work hard for that perfect sculpted physique that he flaunts. After signing Karan Johar's biggest franchise, *Student of the Year 2*, and the parallel lead opposite Hrithik Roshan in Yash Raj Films' untitled project to be directed by Siddharth Anand, he has caught the eye of teenagers, who hope to follow in their idol's footsteps. Tiger is certainly a prime example of how extreme discipline and perseverance can lead to success.

7

Bipasha Basu: Abs-olutely Gorgeous

Her tryst with tinsel town almost unfurled like a Hollywood movie. A clever girl who grew up as a 'tomboy' in a middle-class locality of Kolkata took Bollywood by storm. She was good at studies and quite popular in school, a reason why she was made the head girl. No one would have predicted that this charming girl would one day grow up to become the famous Bollywood actress, fondly called Bips. The same woman, known for her seductive voice, sensuous lips and ability to captivate audiences, is remembered by her classmates as the one who would romp around the colony with a stick in her hands, forever ready to take up the cudgels on behalf of her sisters or friends who felt intimidated by local mischief-makers. She was nicknamed 'Lady Goonda'. Bipasha always had an athletic frame that she worked on constantly with a lot of determination. She has fond recollections of her schooldays and often says, 'I used to be very short as a child and was the class monitor. When tall boys would be up to mischief, I'd jump on their backs during breaks and pull their hair and beat them up.'[1]

However, this brave diva of Bollywood was not always courageous. She did faint while dissecting a laboratory specimen during one of her science classes and thus gave up her dream of becoming a doctor. After that, she switched to commerce and wished to become a chartered accountant. But once again, destiny intervened in 1996, when she was spotted by none other than former Miss India and supermodel Mehr Jessia in a city hotel. She was just in her teens then but Mehr must have seen a spark and suggested to Bipasha to consider modelling as a profession. This changed her life forever. She won the Godrej Cinthol Supermodel Contest organized by Ford and went on to represent India at the Ford Models Supermodel of the World contest in Miami, an international contest established by Eileen Ford in 1980 to discover new talent for the fashion industry. The winner of the final event usually receives a whopping $250,000 modelling contract with Ford Models. Bipasha not only won the prestigious title but also went on to conquer the world of fashion. For Bipasha, it was not just a big break into the fashion world, it was also an introduction to a whole new world of glitz and glamour.

One of the judges at the Godrej Cinthol Supermodel Contest was Vinod Khanna. He was already on the lookout for a fresh face to launch alongside his son Akshaye Khanna in the movie *Himalay Putra*. Bipasha was then just seventeen and wasn't too sure if she was keen on taking up acting as a career. She declined.

Once back in Kolkata, she was asked by Jaya Bachchan to star opposite her son Abhishek Bachchan in J.P. Dutt's film, *Aakhri Mughal*. However, the film was canned and Dutt changed the script to launch Abhishek Bachchan and Kareena Kapoor in *Refugee*. Bipasha was also offered a role in a film opposite Suniel Shetty, but she was still in two minds and declined the offer. Meanwhile, she got busy with her modelling assignments and appeared on well-known and niche magazine covers and live shows. She was not just chiselled, with the perfect muscle tone, she also had a fluidity to her demeanour that made her stand out when she finally descended on tinsel town.

In 2001, Bipasha took the plunge and made her foray into Bollywood movies with director duo Abbas–Mustan's romantic thriller *Ajnabee*. The film starred Akshay Kumar and Kareena Kapoor along with Bobby Deol and Bipasha Basu. Bipasha's performance was highly lauded, and she went on to win the Filmfare Award for best female debut.

In 2002, Bipasha consolidated her position in Bollywood with Vikram Bhatt's thriller, *Raaz*. Critics not just praised her fine performance as an actress, but also her fit and sexy frame. She was again nominated for the Filmfare Award for best actress for *Raaz*. The same year her acting prowess was noticed in *Mere Yaar Ki Shaadi Hai*, where she appeared in a supporting role.

The year 2003 began with a bang for Bipasha. Pooja Bhatt's erotic thriller, *Jism* featured the sizzling diva opposite John Abraham. Bollywood was taken by storm. No other actress had that fluid frame to carry off such sensuous and steamy scenes. Film critic Taran Adarsh, former editor of the film website Bollywood Hungama, said, '[T]he real show stealer in *Jism* is Bipasha Basu; her sexy look and seductive deep voice, in contrast with her cold and calculating personality, makes her the most impressive femme fatale since Zeenat Aman and Parveen Babi.'[2] Bipasha was a sensation, just like Sharon Stone had been in *Basic Instinct* with her seductive scenes. She got a Filmfare Award nomination for best villain for *Jism*.

One can't forget the sizzling performance Bipasha gave in Sonu Nigam's music video album *Kismat*. She mesmerized the audience with her song 'Tu' from the album. She also appeared in Jay Sean's music video for 'Stolen'. Soon, she was getting busier by the day. In 2004, she had four releases, all of which performed moderately and drew mixed reviews. In

2005, she featured in *Barsaat* alongside Bobby Deol and Priyanka Chopra. Bipasha then wanted to diversify her acting portfolio. She was quickly roped into the Tamil film *Sachein*, which was a hit, and then went on to star in Prakash Jha's *Apaharan*.

Being Called Overweight by a Film Magazine

While doing *Apaharan* in 2005, Bipasha realized she had to give more time to fitness and bodybuilding. In her own words to *Mumbai Mirror* journalist Maike Steuer in 2013, 'When I started out as a model, I took things for granted. Because I bagged work thanks to my looks, I didn't give my body any importance.'[3] These were years when Bipasha was a couch potato and admits she had no strict diet plan. She would eat almost anything and everything. In 2005, a tabloid ran a story calling Bipasha fat, which came as a blow to Bips. She said, 'I am famous. How can I be fat?'[4]

She decided to challenge herself and get fit. In her frenzy to shed flab, she took to jogging on the roads and on the treadmill like a maniac, but without any professional help.

The Impact of Exercising Incorrectly

During the shooting of Anees Bazmee's *No Entry*, Bipasha started experiencing excruciating pain in her knees. The pain was so intense she could hardly move her limbs. After several tests, she was diagnosed with osteoarthritis. Bips was shocked. At the age of twenty-four, her world seemed to crumble before her eyes, and she wept for three days as the reality sank in.

Osteoarthritis (OA, or degenerative arthritis) is a joint disease caused by cartilage loss in a joint, which leads to pain and stiffness. 'Being diagnosed with arthritis at an early age made me realize the importance of staying fit,' said Bipasha to *Mumbai Mirror* in 2012.[5] There was a time when she could barely walk, and people around her frightened her by saying she would have to be careful for the rest of her life as she would be unable to dance or do action sequences in movies.

That's when she turned to physiotherapy and began reading up on the complexity of the human body. She realized how different genres of training could target various parts of the body and how wrong exercises could take a severe toll on the bones and muscles. Bipasha's experience is definitely an eye-opener for those who think that just hitting the gym will take care of your fitness regimen. It does not. Planning your workout regimen and diet according to your body type, particularly with a trainer (if you have access to one) is a must, else you will do more harm than good.

Since then, Bipasha has defined 'being fit' in a wholesome way. She says, 'Due to unlimited stress, lifestyle diseases are fast attacking youngsters at a very early age. Hence, you should treat your body as a temple and worship it to remain fit.'[6] After the initial shock, she decided to fight back.

Though her osteoarthritis is now under control due to her holistic lifestyle, she is aware that her foe in this case is strong, and she has to be careful throughout her life to keep osteoarthritis attacks at bay. She firmly believes in the importance of a healthy body and says, 'If you don't have a healthy body, you have nothing.'

Bipasha's Trainer

Bipasha began training under Paul Britto in 2005. They clicked instantly. For Bips, Paul was a godsend. 'He is an angel. My energy levels rarely dip, but if they do, Paul guides me. My regular workout includes a combination of weight training and cardio exercises to boost up my metabolic rates. I come up with a variety of routines that can boost metabolism so that more calories are burnt,' she told *Mumbai Mirror* journalist Maike Steuer in 2013.[7]

Paul helped her get back to shooting full-time the very next year after her diagnosis. She came back with a vengeance and proved her potential as an actress in major releases—*Phir Hera Pheri, Omkara* and *Dhoom 2*. All her films were commercial hits and Bips was praised for the versatile roles. *Phir Hera Pheri* became the ninth-highest-grossing film of the year. As Bianca in *Omkara*, Vishal Bharadwaj's adaptation of Shakespeare's *Othello*, her dance to the song 'Beedi' was lapped up by the public and marked another milestone of her success in the industry. The song sequence revealed her sexy moves, and fit and agile body. For someone with osteoarthritis, it was a challenge to bounce back and dance so fluidly.

In *Dhoom 2*, she looked every inch as gorgeous as she did when she donned her two-piece bikini. The media went gaga over her look. Nikhat Kazmi of the *Times of India* commented: 'Aah, Bipasha! Looks great, brings back the bikini to Bollywood.' She donned her bikini look again with confidence and elan in *Players* (2012) and *Humshakals* (2014).

In 2013, Basu made her foray into Hollywood with the historical romance *The Lovers,* in which she played a Maratha warrior. She followed that by featuring as the host of the television horror series *Darr Sabko Lagta Hai* in 2015.

Bipasha's Training Regimen

Nicknamed Billo Rani (a song from her 2007 release, *Dhan Dhana Dan Goal*), Bipasha is a tall girl at 5 feet 8.5 inches. Her trainer, Paul Britto, compliments her and insists Bips is the fittest among most of her contemporary female stars in Bollywood.

Bipasha not only hits the gym for regular workout sessions but is also passionate about yoga.

She begins her day with 108 rounds of surya namaskar. The sequence of gracefully linked surya namaskars work as a great warm-up routine. This yogic cycle stimulates the entire organ system of the body and makes her fit and healthy, boosting her energy levels and improving awareness.

Bipasha's regular workout is for about two hours daily and includes a combination of cardio and yoga. This has helped her achieve a toned figure and also increased her muscle mass.

Bipasha combines plenty of modern exercise techniques to keep monotony at bay, and her trainer has devised a workout regimen that is geared towards her goal. Bipasha explains, 'For the longest time, Indian women have been okay with being curvy. But I think the modern Indian woman needs to get toned. I don't endorse being thin. Anorexia and bulimia are a reality in India because everybody wants to be thin. A 90-60-90 (a perfectly shaped body in terms of global measurements) body stat is bullshit. It's about the glow that you have on your face and the happiness you exude.'

While many of her contemporaries worked really hard for the size-zero look, Bipasha instead went ahead and popularized curves! 'My mantra is to love yourself and work out for your heart and soul. It has done wonders for me,' she says.[8]

When asked about changing her look for a role, Bipasha has been known to state, 'I would never put on 20 kg and mess up my system because a role demands it. Bollywood doesn't offer you roles that get you an Oscar anyway. Tom Hanks can do it in Hollywood, not us.'

Bipasha's Fitness Video

A staunch advocate of overall fitness of body and soul, Bipasha launched her first fitness DVD in 2010, titled *Love Yourself*. It emphasized on being strong, healthy, and loving one's self. In 2014, she launched another set of three DVDs on fitness, titled *Fit and Fabulous*. This was intended to initiate and lead fitness enthusiasts through a set of sure-shot circuit-training routines that combine upper- and lower-body sculpting moves to burn fat even faster. This fast-paced workout regimen for both beginners and advanced fitness enthusiasts can transform one's body from fat to fit in sixty days.

Bipasha's Daily Gym Training

A typical day for Bipasha begins with a glass of warm water with lime, the surya-namaskar cycle and then hitting the gym.

Monday

On Monday, her workout regimen is aimed at toning her upper body. The upper-body intensive exercises help tone and sculpt back muscles, chest and shoulders. Her line-up consists of:

- 2–3 reps of chin-ups (5 sets)
- 8–10 reps of one-arm dumb-bell rows, superset[9] with 1 dumb-bell bicep curl (3 sets)
- 8–10 reps of face pulls. Superset with seated bent-over rear-delt raises (3 sets)
- 5–7 reps of alternating renegade rows (3 sets)

Tuesday

She devotes the second day of the week to an abdomen workout. This exercise regimen helps lose belly fat and develop strong core muscles and flat abs. Bipasha begins with a series of exercises that include stability-ball pelvic tilt-crunch, followed by rotating plank, arm pull-over straight-leg crunch, the matrix, nose-to-knee crunch, prone oblique roll and concludes with back extension rear leg-raise.

Wednesday

On Wednesday, Bipasha concentrates on her legs with a lower-body workout.

- Leg extensions, superset with lying leg-curls: 15–20 reps (3–4 sets)
- Lying leg-curls, superset with leg extensions: 15–20 reps (3–4 sets)

- Wide-stance barbell squats: 110 reps (10 sets)
- Seated calf-raises: 15 reps (4 sets)
- Front barbell squats: 8–10 reps (4 sets)
- Body-weight reverse lunges: 12–15 reps, alternating (4 sets)
- One-leg barbell squat, superset with jump squat: 12–15 reps per leg (3 sets)
- Jump squats, superset with one-leg barbell squat: 12–15 reps (3 sets)
- Stiff-legged barbell dead-lifts: 12–15 reps (3 sets)
- Lying leg-curls, superset with walking lunges: 15–20 reps (3 sets)
- Body-weight walking lunges, superset with lying leg-curls: 12–15 reps per leg (3 sets)
- Speed squats with resistance band: 2 sets

It is no wonder then that Bipasha has some of the sexiest legs in Bollywood.

Thursday
Bipasha reserves her Thursdays for a gluteus maximus (butt) workout.

She begins with squats and moves on to single-leg dead-lift which work the glutes more than regular dead-lifts.

Lunges are next in line. Lunges are an excellent exercise that target all of the gluteus muscles, especially the gluteus maximus. Static lunges, like forward or reverse lunges, are the most common form.

Bips also does cardio exercises to reduce body fat and build strong muscles. Climbing stairs—whether it's ten flights of stairs or the StairMaster at the gym—at a steady pace helps firming and shaping the butt. She also sprints because sprinting requires power and explosiveness that comes from the glutes and legs.

Friday

On Fridays, Bipasha works on her upper body.

Her regimen includes:

- Dumb-bell bench presses, superset with dips: 8–10 reps (3 sets)
- Dips, triceps version: 10–12 reps (3 sets)
- Dumb-bell one-arm shoulder presses, superset with standing dumb-bell upright rows: 10–12 reps (3 sets)
- Incline push-ups: 8–15 reps (3 sets)
- Lying dumb-bell tricep extensions: 6–8 reps (3 sets)

Saturday

On the sixth day of the week, Bipasha repeats her abdomen or gluteus maximus workouts, alternating between the two. She takes rest on Sunday, staying away from her strict exercise routine. With a rigorous regimen like this, one is bound to notice immediate changes in their body and push further. However, Bipasha never tries to overdo things as she is haunted by the fear of injuries or ailments, something that she has experienced first-hand. After she damaged her left knee due to excessive running on the treadmill, she took care to space out her rigorous cardio workouts. In a fifty-minute session, she devotes twenty minutes on the treadmill, ten minutes on the elliptical trainer and twenty minutes on the rowing machine.

Discipline

Bipasha puts emphasis on discipline and says, 'If you want to lead a healthy lifestyle, you need to be fit. To set up an effective fitness routine, you must have a disciplined approach.' She is also vehemently opposed to quick-fix solutions like having slimming pills or opting for crash diets. They only have a temporary effect on the body but in the long run do more harm than good. Only a well-devised regular exercise regimen eventually works wonders. In this context, she says one should change the workout format daily to keep it more interesting and enjoyable. She advises drinking plenty of water and staying away from junk and deep-fried food to cleanse the internal system and get rid of harmful toxins. A well-hydrated body gives the skin a natural lustre. She says, 'Your body is what you eat, so keep strict vigilance on your diet.'

Bipasha's Diet Plan

Though a self-proclaimed 'born foodie', Bipasha is very conscious of what she eats and what she should abstain from. She is very fond of fish and includes both fish and nuts in her diet as they are rich in omega-3 fatty acids. She also has plenty of fresh green leafy vegetables, sprouts and fruits for that glowing skin. Bipasha is a morning person, and her day starts early.

Early Morning
- A glass of warm water with lime.
- A handful of almonds soaked overnight and a cup of green tea without sugar. Sometimes, she substitutes her green tea with wheatgrass shots.

Breakfast
- An hour after her rigorous workout session, Bips has a sumptuous breakfast.
- It consists of six egg whites, brown-bread toast, mushroom, porridge and fruits.

A heavy and balanced breakfast provides energy to sail through the day.

It also jump-starts the body's metabolism and helps digestion and absorption of nutrients in the body.

Lunch

- Bipasha likes to keep her lunch small and simple. Though boiled rice is a staple food in any Bengali household, Bipasha abstains from consuming it for lunch. She loves rice but has stopped eating it since *No Entry* (2005). She switched to wheat, which contains more protein, minerals and fibre than rice. She says, 'I think wheat is great. You mix wheat with bajra so you can have bajre ki roti or soya rotis.'[10]
- She has two chapattis with a bowl of dal and mixed vegetables cooked in olive oil. She is very fastidious about her cooking medium and insists on using only olive oil for all types of food preparations.
- However, once in a while she does enjoy her puris and parathas as well. Her mantra is: Eat everything, but in moderation, and burn those extra calories through simple exercises.

Desserts

Bipasha has a sweet tooth and is very fond of desserts. She staunchly believes one should not starve the body.

'I'm a true Bengali; I love mithai. And if you have a balanced diet most of the time, you can reward yourself and satisfy your cravings once in a while.'[11]

Bipasha's Tips to Attain Washboard Abs

To have sexy abs, Bipasha feels the following superfoods are the best.

Oats with cinnamon: Oats are a great way to start the day. They keep the tummy full for a longer time, while cinnamon has natural thermionic properties and aids metabolism.

Grapefruit: Grapefruit helps lower insulin levels, promoting weight loss in the process. It also helps increase metabolism.

Red peppers: Peppers contain capsaicin, which burns stubborn fat.

Almonds: Rich in protein, almonds help keep the tummy full for a long time and boost the metabolism.

Salmon: Salmon is loaded with omega-3 fatty acids, which is beneficial for fat loss.

Avocado: Avocados contain healthy fat that provides essential energy to the body.

Blueberries: Blueberries are loaded with antioxidants. Low in sugar, this low-calorie fruit is a good snacking option.

Green tea: Green tea is rich in antioxidants and helps cleanse the body.

Chicken: Chicken is a great source of lean protein and helps weight loss.

Sweet potato: Sweet potatoes stabilize blood-sugar levels and aid metabolism.

Conclusion

Bipasha is a workaholic and she confesses, 'I am active even on bad days; it's tough to pin me down. People ask me if I am a morning or a night person. I am an all-the-time person. I like drinking coffee but I do it with lots of milk because my energy levels are high even without caffeine. You could call me Obelix, except I don't have a belly.' While green tea helps Bipasha cut down on additional calories, coffee with milk gives her energy. Her fantastic metabolism means she doesn't put on weight on her tummy. However, she prefers skimmed or soya milk.

Now that's what Bipasha Basu is for you. A down-to-earth, no-nonsense person with a zest for life. And surely a body to die for.

8

Shahid Kapoor: Fiery and Fit

His Bollywood Story

Shahid Kapoor is a powerhouse of energy, passion and playfulness. He's not just a phenomenal dancer but also an emotive actor.

The son of actors Pankaj Kapur and Neelima Azeem, Shahid saw his parents separate when he was three years old, which he confesses made him unhappy as a child. However, it never deterred him from single-mindedly pursuing his career and achieving tremendous triumphs on the way. Extremely talented, Shahid is a versatile actor who can play a wide variety of roles and give performances ranging from light comedy to passionate drama. He's also one of the best dancers in Bollywood.

Shahid made his film debut in 2003 in the romantic comedy *Ishq Vishk*, in a lead role and won the Filmfare Award for best male debut. His next notable performance was in Sooraj Barjatya's family drama *Vivaah* (2006), which was a high grosser at the box office. In 2007, he played a troubled businessman in Imtiaz Ali's *Jab We Met*, which went on to become a huge hit and earned him a nomination for the Filmfare Award for best actor. In 2013, he starred in the action film *R . . . Rajkumar*, which was a commercial success. In Vishal Bhardwaj's *Haider* (2014), the audience loved Shahid's powerful and intense rendering of Hamlet's character. This earned him Filmfare's best actor award. In 2016, he again displayed some excellent acting skills when he played a junkie singer in the crime thriller *Udta Punjab*. He won the Filmfare Critics' Award for best actor for this role. He then featured in Vishal Bharadwaj's *Rangoon* alongside Kangana Ranaut and Saif Ali Khan.

His most recent film *Padmaavat* is a fictionalized period drama about the life of the legendary queen Rani Padmavati (played by Deepika Padukone) and her husband Rana Rawal Ratan Singh, ruler of Mewar (played by Shahid).

In spite of a few flops here and there, Shahid has retained his popularity as a talented actor and fabulous dancer. His attractive and charming looks combined with a well-toned, muscular physique make him very popular with the youth. He is married to Mira Rajput, with whom he has a daughter. He is a dedicated supporter of several charitable organizations and has adopted three villages to support NDTV's Greenathon initiative, which promotes environmental consciousness and has improved electricity supply to rural areas.

However, Shahid's breakthrough performance with which he first burst on to the scene was his double role in Vishal Bharadwaj's *Kaminey* (2009). Dominated by the dark and dangerous world of the drug mafia and gang wars, this movie leaves you on the edge of your seat as you are taken on a rollercoaster ride of fast-paced action scenes and powerful performances.

Throughout the movie, Shahid looked like a hunk, bulging biceps straining through his grungy T-shirts. It was quite a transformation from the sweet, boyish looks he had sported in romance films such as *Ishq Vishk, Fida, Chup Chup Ke, Dil Maange More* and *Deewane Huye Paagal*. He suddenly went from a lean chocolate boy to a beefy badass.

Kaminey Workout Secrets

Shahid's trainer for *Kaminey,* Abbas Ali, was the man responsible for his shockingly fabulous transformation. This 2014 winner of the Men's Health award for best personal trainer in India shares the precious secrets that catapulted Shahid permanently into the 'muscle club' of Bollywood.

Abbas says, 'The role required him to look rough and raw. Basically, like a rugged, full-grown man. So we put him on something known as combined training which is based on eleven elements of fitness. He went through six to eight months of intensive training and fitness workouts. The training was a combination of MMA (mixed martial-arts), parkour, callisthenics, yoga and strength conditioning. Strength training is something bodybuilders do. But we incorporated something known as strength conditioning which is more on the lines of endurance training.'[1]

Training for *Kaminey*

Giant Sets: Upper-body Routine

Set 1 (5 sets with 1-minute rest in between)
- 10 flat bench-presses
- 10 chin-ups
- 10 dead-lifts
- 10 lateral raises

Set 2 (5 sets with 1-minute rest in between)
- 10 incline dumb-bell presses
- 10 bent-over barbell rows
- 10 overhead presses
- 10 shrugs

Set 3
- 50 seated rows
- 50 machine flyes
- 50 high-pulls
- 50 rear-delt flyes
- Cool-down: Upper-body stretch

Giant Sets: Lower-body Routine

Set 1 (4 sets with 2-minute rest in between)
- 15 leg extensions
- 15 squats
- 15 leg curls
- 15 standing calf-raises

Set 2 (4 sets with 2-minute rest in between)
- 50 leg presses
- 50 stiff-leg dead-lifts
- 50 step-ups
- 50 seated calf-raises

Cool-down: Lower-body stretch

Functional Training: Upper-body Split

Round 1 (5 rounds without rest)
- 50 clean and presses
- 50 sit-ups

- 12 chin-ups
- 10 hanging leg-raises
- 50 push-ups

Round 2 (4 rounds without rest)
- 50 overheard presses
- 50 dead-lifts

Cool-down: Stretch

Shoulder, Legs and Abs Split

Round 1 (3 to 5 sets without rest)
- 50 thrust-squats with dumb-bells
- 50 hanging leg-raises

Round 2 (3 to 5 sets without rest)
- 50 sumo dead-lifts
- 50 sit-ups

Round 3 (3 to 5 sets without rest)
- 50 push-presses or clean and presses
- 50 reverse crunches

Round 4 (3 to 5 sets without rest)
- 50 Russian swings (hip and knee extension)
- 50 crunches

Cool-down: Full-body stretch

Shahid did strength training twice a week for muscle hypertrophy and relied on functional training twice a week to improve his muscle endurance and muscle quality.

To prepare for the memorable and high-powered scene of Shahid running with the horses, high-intensity interval training was included in his training to enhance his running skills and form.

Dancing Dervish

A product of Shiamak Davar's dance academy in Mumbai, Shahid is among the famous choreographer's favourite students. Shahid also has a lot of respect for Shiamak Davar, 'Shiamak has been a friend to me. I learnt the fundamentals of professional conduct and dance from him. His contribution to my journey is huge and I'll always be grateful to him.'[2]

Shahid is extremely passionate about dancing. In fact, like Hrithik, his performances were first noticed due to his high-voltage dancing skills.

The power-packed live performances Shahid gives for award ceremonies and shows have earned him a huge fan following, as have his memorable dancing moves in films.

The film that really highlighted these skills was the dance-driven film *Chance Pe Dance*. Choreography is the highlight of the film and the dance directors gave Shahid some challenging steps to perform. And because of his immense flexibility and fitness levels, Shahid performed with effortless ease and grace. He also sported chiselled washboard abs in this film. In fact, the look required of him was very different from that in *Kaminey*. Abbas Ali says of that period, 'Shahid didn't have a muscular body. I was training him only for fitness. He didn't want the perfect body of *Kaminey*, because in that movie he plays a guy who comes from the streets and thus does not work out in a high-tech gym.'[3] But for *Chance Pe Dance*, he needed a sculpted body. So Abbas changed his workouts to bring about this highly enhanced, cosmetically appealing look. He focused on flexibility and muscle endurance to give him the extra edge required for his dance performances in the film. Incidentally, this was also the film where Shahid first sported an eight-pack, acquired under the guidance of Abbas. He had to undergo functional training which included a lot of sports to strengthen his core and keep his body agile at the same time. 'He would train for an hour every day for five days a week. We made sure that his body stayed flexible and did not harden up so he could dance well in the film,'[4] says Ali. Shahid had to undergo almost a year of hardcore training to achieve the desired look for this film. One advantage while developing this look was that Shahid had already gained lean muscle while training for *Kaminey*. So Abbas planned out his new training schedule within a week after *Kaminey*. 'I always say you are the product of your training and lifestyle . . . And if you want to look like an athlete, you need to understand how athletes train and eat . . . I took the best of every art/training to get him in this shape.'[5] Not only was Shahid required to look his best, he also needed stamina, endurance and flexibility for the role. Such high expectations needed that hard-core backup training.

Given below is the 'workout from hell', as Abbas calls it.

The Workout from Hell: Functional Training Sample 1

- 50 jump pull-ups
- 200-metre run
- 50 overheard presses
- 200-metre run
- 50 dead-lifts
- 200-metre run
- 50 hanging leg-raises
- 200-metre run
- 50 push-presses

- 200-metre run
- 50 pull-ups
- 200-metre run
- 50 high-pulls
- 200-metre run
- 50 bar dips
- 200-metre run
- 50 Russian swings
- 200-metre run
- 50 burpees
- 200-metre run
- 1 round without rest

Cool-down: Stretch

The Delta Force: Functional Training Sample 2

This is what gave Shahid his well-balanced deltoids

Round 1 (5 sets without rest)
- 10 clean and presses
- 10 overheard presses
- 10 high-pulls
- 10 curl-presses
- 10 dumb-bell shrugs

Round 2 (5 sets without rest)
- 50 lateral raises

- 50 upright rows
- 50 rear-deltoid flyes
- 50 barbell shrugs

Cool-down: Stretch

Sports and Parkour Conditioning

This was a part of his agility, flexibility, coordination and balance training where Shahid did vaulting, precision jumps, jumping hurdles, lower-body drills, etc.

Yoga

Ali incorporated the best of yoga poses in the training for core stability, flexibility and mental endurance.

Metabolic Conditioning

Running, skipping, sprinting, cycling, burpees, box jumps etc., were done to achieve the athletic look.

Diet

Shahid's diet too underwent slight changes. Being a vegetarian, there was not much that the nutritionists or trainers could change. If he had been a non-vegetarian, he could have switched to eating leaner protein like white fish instead of chicken. But as Abbas says, 'Shahid doesn't even eat eggs so first-class protein which is required to build lean muscle was not there. White carbs like white potatoes, pasta and white rice were removed from his diet. We added brown carbs like brown rice, sweet potatoes and oats instead.'

To make sure he added or maintained muscle mass while keeping his body fat to a minimum, it was extremely important that Shahid had a calculated nutrition plan to fall back on.

Vivid, Vibrant and Vegetarian

As a staunch vegetarian, Shahid's prime focus in his diet is to derive maximum nutrients that will provide a high level of energy needed to sustain the intensity and strength required for his workouts. His nutritionists ensure that his daily meals are packed with all essential nutrients and nine amino acids. The amino acids, which are a combination of leucine, isoleucine and valine, help in recovering after intense workouts. Shahid's diet is therefore a balanced mix of low-fat tofu, paneer, soy, brown rice, quinoa, lots of fresh fruits and vegetables.

But surprisingly his diet comprises some delectable and varied dishes. This comes as a surprise when one thinks of the bland and boring meals actors generally have. When Shahid first met Samir Jaura, the reputed Bollywood fitness trainer, to get into shape for *Padmaavat*, he told him, 'Sam, I need to look like a prince. You need to help me with my diet. I'm a vegetarian.' Samir replied that he was a vegetarian himself, so he could help him. 'So ours was a superb combination and we bonded on the spot. I sorted out a veg. diet for him that was a fabulous combination of high proteins, carbs and fibre. He loved it,' confides Samir.

Truly, Shahid's meals were bursting with choices. Also, Samir reveals that once he had outlined all the options available to the actor, his wife Mira took over and rigorously monitored all his meals. 'All his meals were home-cooked and prepared under the supervision of his wife,' he says

Breakfast: Oatmeal cooked with skimmed milk and almonds, raisins and walnuts (1 bowl)/brown-rice idlis (4–5) with green coriander chutney/2 green moong dal cheelas with mint chutney/millet upma (1 bowl)/2 soya toasts with peanut butter/2 vegetable and soya cutlets with green chutney/brown-rice poha (1 bowl) with a glass of fresh fruit juice and a bowl of fruit.

Midday Snack: A whey protein shake.

Lunch: Kaala channa biryani (made with brown rice) + a bowl of raita and cucumber salad/matar paneer made with low-fat paneer (1 bowl) + green moong dal (1 bowl) + 2 rice-flour rotis/besan kadhi with brown rice (1 bowl) + cabbage ki sabzi + 2 rice-flour rotis/rajma (1 bowl) with brown rice (1 bowl)—this is Shahid's all-time favourite/couscous (1 bowl) with salad and beans topped with a cucumber and dill yoghurt dressing/Stir-fried veggies: bok choy, broccoli, asparagus and mushrooms with tofu (1 bowl) along with 4–5 steamed dim-sum made with wholewheat flour.

Evening snack: Sweet potatoes chaat (1 bowl)/boiled green moong dal salad/peanut salad/4–5 brown-rice dhoklas/2 yam and veg. cutlets with mint chutney (yam is high in fibre)/chickpea salad + protein shake

Dinner: Sukhi moong ki dal (1 bowl) + low-fat matar paneer (1 bowl) + 2 wholewheat rotis + chickpea salad/2 wholewheat pita breads within 4–5 shallow-fried falafels/soya-granules pulao made with brown rice + raita + green moong salad/dal makhni (cream substituted with milk to give the dal its creamy texture) + gobhi matar + brown rice (1 bowl)/veg. sushi with a clear veg. soup

All of Shahid's meals were cooked in olive oil, which was used sparingly. As Shahid loves spicy food, spices were not eliminated from his diet completely but reduced. Salt too was moderately used.

Throughout the diet, Samir ensured that Shahid got a lot of protein from sources such as pulses, paneer, tofu, yoghurt, rajma. His complex carbs came from rice flour, wholewheat, millet etc., and his fibre and vitamins from vegetables, salads and fruits. Sugar was not allowed but Shahid kept up his blood sugar from fruits that have a high content of natural sugars or fructose. So all in all, Shahid's diet was well balanced and the quantities proportionate to the energy he was expending on his daily workouts.

Samir gave him a cheat day every fifteen days, during which he was allowed to order food or eat in restaurants and gorge on pastries, cakes and brownies. Shahid is a coffee addict so Samir allowed him his two cups or shots of black coffee in a day. His water intake was fixed at 5 litres a day. Samir maintains that if more than this quantity of water is consumed, it can be harmful for the body; the excess water flushes out essential minerals and vitamins from the body.

As Shahid is a pure vegetarian, he does not consume any vitamins or supplements that are made with gelatinous capsules or have animal fat content.

Pre-Body Shots Diet

Forty days before the close-up for the body shots were required to be taken for *Padmaavat*, Shahid was put on a stringent diet. He was allowed only 50 to 70 g brown or black rice with broccoli, asparagus and beans along with pulses and rajma for protein, four to five times in a day. Half a teaspoon of olive oil was used throughout the day for cooking his meals. Twenty days before the shoot, salt was eliminated completely. Also, his favourite beverage coffee was denied to him. There were no cheat days during this period.

But like a thorough professional, Shahid complied without any complaints and followed his diet religiously.

Workout Regimen for a 'Warrior King'

Shahid works out regularly and keeps his body in good shape. Samir reveals, 'I enjoyed working with Shahid as he is very interested in training. He goes into a lot of detail and asks a lot of questions regarding the training. He's a fitness fan.'

Samir reveals that Shahid's body has very good muscle memory and muscle maturity as he's been working out consistently for the past fifteen to sixteen years. But he adds that although this definitely helps, the look required for every film changes. So both the trainer and the actor have to put in considerable effort to achieve that look. 'I have to use my time training with the actor in a very focused manner. I can't waste time experimenting with different workouts. It's all very structured and I have to work around the look that is needed for the film. Shahid enjoys training so he was open to whatever I had planned for him,' he says, adding, 'You have to make sure his body looks proportionate and aesthetically appealing. Also the actor has to be very committed and give his 100 per cent to achieve the look. That way Shahid is a perfectionist, just like Farhan.'

In fact, just like Farhan, Shahid's body type too, is ectomorphic. But he's also half mesomorph, which is an advantage. Mesomorph body types are characterized by athletic, strong, compact and naturally lean bodies. They could be called 'genetically gifted' and also have excellent posture. In men, the shoulders are wider than their hips. They are natural athletes and tend to be lean and muscular without much effort. They are generally of medium build. The world's leading tennis players and bodybuilders fall into this group: Andre Agassi, Sylvester Stallone and Arnold Schwarzenegger.

With all these positives, Shahid had an advantage. Or rather only half the advantage as he's also half ectomorph. Slim-boned and long-limbed ectomorph body types are usually prevalent among models and supermodels. They tend to be more on the skinny side and find it difficult to put on weight, with little body fat and muscle mass and high metabolisms. Also they have difficulty gaining muscle mass and body weight. Shahid being a combination of the two was guided accordingly by Samir. To achieve the targets required for the role, Samir put Shahid through a number of different training programmes over the course of a year.

Initially Shahid went through a boot camp training regimen. Samir would set up a training camp on the beach next to his house with a lot of training equipment that he'd bring with him, including ladders, sand bags, tyres, slam balls, cones and battle ropes.

Shahid then went through functional training, endurance training, agility training, strength training, kettlebell training and CrossFit training.

Functional training is more related to purposeful training for sports, but it has been successfully incorporated into fitness workouts as well. It involves exercises that allow one to be more flexible. To build his body, Shahid focused on weight-bearing activities that targeted the core muscles of the abdomen and lower back. This also provided stability, strength, endurance, power and flexibility, improving basic movements like walking and running.

Endurance training helped Shahid improve cardiovascular, respiratory and muscular endurance. He could build up tolerance levels to withstand stress, pain and fatigue.

Speed and agility training workouts made sure that Shahid focused on leg and core muscles as well as tendons.

Strength training was used to build and strengthen muscle mass while the kettlebell made sure his joints were tougher and less prone to injury. These were mostly whole-body movement exercises that also strengthened the tendons and ligaments.

Shahid's CrossFit training regimen included various functional movements performed at high-intensity levels.

Samir's Advice for Beginners

- Perform your workouts with the help of a professional. Also plan your workouts under such guidance.
- Assess your body type and then focus accordingly on the workouts that will suit you best.
- Cross-check or look into the credibility of your trainer. They should have proper training credentials or qualifications necessary for training people.

- Try and play a sport that involves physical activity. This will keep the body fit and flexible.
- Eat a balanced and healthy diet. Avoid fast food. Eat more home-cooked meals comprising basic pulses, vegetables, wholewheat grains and fruits. If you're non vegetarian, eating eggs with yolks is fine till your early thirties—unless one is clinically obese or facing cholesterol issues.
- Say no to recreational drugs like smoking etc. Also alcohol is bad for the body, so try to avoid it.
- Try to work out regularly to build muscle memory and muscle maturity over a period of time, slowly but surely.
- You must eat a supporting diet that corresponds with the intensity of your workouts.
- Seven to eight hours of sleep and adequate rest is recommended for the body. This helps the body recover from any wear and tear of muscles during workouts and also builds or strengthens muscle mass.
- Sixteen to seventeen years is the perfect age to start working out.

Samir says, ultimately, it is the level of your commitment and dedication which will help you achieve your fitness goals. For the movie *Padmaavat*,

Samir and Shahid were able to achieve the physique demanded by the role. In fact, Samir says, 'When I went to take a look at the monitor to see how Shahid's shots had come out, I said "Shahid, you are looking like Brad Pitt. And I'm not joking about this."'

Shahid's Daily Workout Routine

Shahid's fitness levels can be credited to his dedicated and disciplined training programme. He is a self-proclaimed fitness freak who believes in exposing his body to a range of fitness activities and techniques to achieve the desired result.

He has been training with Abbas since his *Chup Chup Ke* days. Since then, as far as his physique is concerned, Shahid has gotten better. From a lean, sculpted frame, he has gone on to achieve a more chiselled, brawny and muscular physique that has stood him in good stead for all the films he has starred in.

Shahid works out six days a week and has a rigorous regimen that exercises each part of his body. This ensures he remains ripped and lean. As advised by Abbas, Shahid does a mix of cardio and strength-training exercises. Shahid also practises yoga, martial arts, swimming, running on the treadmill, and does weight training.

Monday, Wednesday, Friday

First set (5 sets of each exercise with 8 reps)
- Flat bench-presses
- Chin-ups
- Dead-lifts
- Lateral raises

Second set (5 sets of each exercise with 8 to 12 reps)
- Incline dumb-bell presses
- Bent-over barbell rows
- Overheard presses

Third set (5 sets of each exercise repeated 8 to 12 times)
- Seated rows
- Chest flyes
- High-pulls
- Dumb-bell rear-deltoid flyes

Tuesday, Thursday, Saturday

First set (4 sets of each exercise with 12 to 15 reps)
- Leg extensions
- Squats
- Leg curls
- Standing calf-raises
- Leg presses

- Stiff-leg dead-lifts
- Step-ups
- Seated calf-raises

Shahid's Basic Diet Plan

As Shahid is a staunch vegetarian, his meals are centred around lots of veggies and fruits. He has a lot of beans, spinach, broccoli and other green vegetables. He ensures he has five to six small meals a day. He also focuses on eating the right pre- and post-workout meals for sustaining his intense workouts. He feels that the number of meals is directly proportional to the intensity of the workouts.

A demanding training schedule should definitely be accompanied by a healthy nutritious diet. Carbs, proteins and fats should be properly balanced in the food intake. To this end, he makes sure he has a healthy breakfast and avoids fried foods and soft drinks. He concentrates on having a high-protein diet which is low in carbs and fat.

To enhance his muscles, Shahid relies on protein supplements including creatine and whey protein. He loves having protein pancakes with stevia and maple syrup, a chocolate mush made with casein protein, etc. So Shahid looks for innovative meals that are packed with protein and healthy alternatives to sugar and fat.

Conclusion

Shahid Kapoor is an actor who has worked very hard to reach where he has, not only in his career, but also his physical appearance. It was quite early in his career that he took to the route of fitness to enhance his body image. It is true that *Kaminey* propelled him to achieve those rugged looks but since then he has made every effort to maintain and build upon it. With his dancing talents added to his now-spectacular physique, it is no wonder he is quite a heart-throb!

9

John Abraham: Body of Work

Over the years, when there has been a need to define the ideal male body, people have repeatedly turned to Michelangelo's David. It seemed like every man in the 1980s and 1990s wished to have a figure like the masterpiece of the great sculptor. David is thought to have the perfect body, and men down the ages have tried to emulate that physical perfection, going to any length in the quest for precision.

In Bollywood, the idea of a handsome man has seen a massive change over the years. In the 1930s and 1940s—decades when pioneering film directors were trying to figure out ways to establish an independent Indian role model, despite the overbearing presence of European and Hollywood movies everywhere—we had the Chaplinesque Raj Kapoor or even the flamboyant Dev Anand, our answer to Hollywood's Gregory Peck. They all portrayed characters who had hearts of gold, ready to save a damsel in distress and even punch and kick a villain or two. They were chivalrous in love, yet followed the diktats of society and led normal lives, despite their heroic deeds.

The 1950s were earmarked for chocolate-box heroes. We had Dilip Kumar, Raaj Kumar, Rajendra Kumar, Manoj Kumar and Shammi Kapoor, actors we thought of as our desi Elvis Presley, followed, later, in the 1960s, by Jeetendra, Dharmendra and Rajesh Khanna. They all looked adorable and portrayed people who were romantic and chivalrous. This 'romance' genre reached its pinnacle of success with the advent of Rajesh Khanna. The 1970s saw the rise of the 'angry young man', Amitabh Bachchan, in an iconic hero/anti-hero format. But even here, the male lead actors did all the action in full mufti. It was a time when showing bare chests and bare bodies on-screen was left to the 'lecherous villains' who followed young nubile girls greedily. Even 'villains' looked uncouth and comical as they moved around with their sagging paunches. Then there were the arty, aka 'parallel', movies, where Naseeruddin Shah or Om Puri were bare-chested on-screen but represented those hardly in need of an impressive, chiselled body. It took another generation or two for Bollywood heroes to muster enough courage to display their well-toned, muscular bodies on-screen, which has now become the norm. Michelangelo's

David has thus been brought to life and given a cult status by the studly Bollywood heroes.

Since the very beginning of his film career, one actor has always come up as the fittest of his class, not just displaying a sculpted muscular torso, but also seriously embodying the concept of staying fit in his daily life. His interviews have appeared in various newspapers and magazines where he has shared some of his insights as a fitness enthusiast. He is none other than John Abraham, the man whose physique has been utilized to the utmost on the big screen by Bollywood directors.

Bollywood's Portrayal of John's Exceptionally Fit Frame

Take any of his movies—*Paap* (2003), *Jism* (2003), *Lakeer*, *Dhoom* (2004) *Dostana* (2008), *New York* (2009) *Force* (2011), *Shootout At Wadala*, *Madras Cafe*, *Race 2* (2013) *Rocky Handsome*, *Force 2* and *Dishoom* (2016)—John has displayed his eight-pack bare torso and muscular biceps with panache.

In *Aashayein* (2010), he portrayed the character of Rahul, a compulsive gambler diagnosed with lung cancer with only three months left to live. For this role, John had to shed 12 kg to look thin and sickly. Soon after this, he had to regain his weight for his next project—YRF's *New York*. Such weight fluctuations usually have a detrimental effect on the body if not done under strict professional supervision. These days, most actors have to change their look to fit into the skin of the character they are offered to portray, and John has proved his mettle every time he has been challenged by directors.

Nishikanth Kamath's action thriller *Force* was released in 2011 with John in the lead. He looked stunning in his perfectly sculpted muscular body. He outdid Aamir Khan and Shah Rukh Khan's eight-pack abs with ten-pack abs. Girls swooned over the modern-day Adonis's body and boys aspired to look like him.

John's Fitness Mantra

It is not an easy task to look like John Abraham. It took him years of hard work and a dedicated, disciplined and holistic approach to life and work to get where he is today. In an interview for fitness enthusiasts, John said: 'Fitness is like a tripod stand; it has three legs—good food, good sleep and [a] good routine.'[1]

John insists that there is no shortcut to success, and if one really desires a well-sculpted physique, one must work hard and achieve it through constant dedication and discipline. He says, 'For me, going to the gym is a necessity and part of my everyday routine. A committed gym regimen, plus good discipline and a proper diet, will help you attain a great body.'

He has been a fitness enthusiast all his life and going to the gym is as essential as breathing for him. He treats his body as a temple, and in one interview he even said, 'I am pretty much an agnostic . . . so my only religion is my body. I think there's nothing more important than health . . . [and my aim is] to live and die with a six-pack.'[2] He propagates the theory that exercise should be a way of life and not a phase, and says that everyone should do some kind of exercise every day to improve their immunity and keep lifestyle diseases, such as obesity, type II diabetes and even high blood pressure, at bay.

But John realizes that everyone can't hit the gym every day. 'You don't need to go to the gym; just play a sport like football, tennis or squash. Get activity into your daily life. Walk an extra stop instead of taking the bus, take the stairs not the lift, walk around while you're on the phone instead of sitting. All these extra little activities soon add up.'[3]

John is very particular about abstaining from addictive substances such as alcohol, drugs or gutkha. He warns everyone against the use of external stimulants such as growth hormones and steroids to enhance body mass, and advises his fans not to go for these quick-fix solutions. He adds that such unnecessary hormone therapies to build up muscles affect the body and mind in the long run.

John's Scientific Approach to Fitness

The actor follows a strict and disciplined workout regimen and knows exactly which part of his body needs to be worked on and when. He has an ecto-mesomorph body, i.e. his body can easily fluctuate between being incredibly lean and very muscular. Males with ecto-mesomorph body have broad shoulders, narrow waists, ankles and wrists, and a 'V' shape of the torso.

Standing tall at 6 feet, John weighs 94 kg, with a 36–inch waist and 21-inch biceps.

John believes that just effort is not enough to build a perfect body. A scientific approach is necessary, and hence one must learn more about one's body type before planning a workout schedule. Each body has different requirements. While working on the movie *Dostana*, the actor realized that all exercises do not suit him.

Just going to a gym and lifting weights for hours does not help build muscles. In fact, chances of damaging muscles and joints increase manifold if a workout is done without prior knowledge of technique, or proper supervision. Workout sessions, according to John, should be efficient and precise.

Sculpting the body is not magic, and one should take a slow and steady approach.

A quick reduction or addition in muscle mass can have a harmful effect on the body. The outer skin layer can lose its elasticity if it is expanded or contracted too fast or too often, and can lead to permanent stretch marks on the body.

A Peek into John's Diet Plan

He eats a simple, balanced diet, which is high in nutrients, to get the right amount of calories required for his body. John never supports fad or crash diets. These don't provide enough nourishment to the body and wreak havoc on the metabolic system, leading to fatigue and loss of vital muscle tissue. In fact, starving only leads to hankering for more food.

What works, according to John, is eating the right food in the right quantity and then burning the calories by working out. John never goes for ready-to-eat (loaded with saturated trans fats and preservatives) popular food items or anything that is deep-fried, oily or greasy. He prefers to munch on an apple or a slice of papaya to satiate his cravings (which seldom occur).

John says if one invests 60 per cent of one's energy in selecting a sensible diet and burns 40 per cent of the accumulated energy, it is possible to achieve that sculptured look. He insists that even if you don't have time to exercise, eating the right food at the right time can have a positive impact on the body. In his words, 'When you eat right, everything about you is better, especially your skin and hair!'[4]

For him, eggs are the best sources of protein, and he believes everyone should include them in their regular diet to build strong muscles. He also suggests including fruits in breakfast in any form to boost energy levels early in the day.

John is very particular about the rule that a wholesome breakfast keeps one going, and never misses his breakfast even when he has a hectic schedule. According to him, skipping breakfast is a common mistake and can have a detrimental effect on the body. The actor refuses to buy the logic that many people do not get time to have breakfast. In such cases, he suggests, one can wake up an hour earlier to eat or prepare something the previous night.

John has his carbohydrates early on as they provide energy for the rest of the day, and the body also gets adequate time to burn them off. This decreases the chances of fat accumulation. If you have a heavy breakfast, you won't snack between meals.

He says, 'Rather than looking at how many calories you get from your meals, look at the nutritional value of what you are eating. The natural sugars that you get from a fruit are obviously better for you than the empty calories in refined sweets. Consume everything from salts to carbs [rice, pasta, potatoes, bread], but in measured, sensible proportions.'[5]

How John Fights His Food Cravings and Chocolate Temptations

John stresses the importance of fighting temptation with moderation. He relates an incident when he was offered piping hot samosas and gulab jamuns on the sets of a movie, which he was tempted to eat, but resisted the urge and walked away. He confesses, 'Even fitness enthusiasts have weaknesses. I love chocolate, yet I keep indulgences to a minimum. There's nothing wrong with an occasional treat, but "occasional" doesn't mean every day!'

This disciplined actor also doesn't believe in cheat days. 'I don't have a cheat day. It's not about a day, it's my lifestyle. So, when there are good things available to eat, why should I go out of the way to eat something bad? I haven't had a cheat day in the last twenty years,' he adds.

John has also been a staunch supporter of the PETA (People for Ethical Treatment of Animals) movement and avoids meat, but eats fish and egg whites to fulfil his protein requirements. He also supplements his diet with whey shakes and protein bars to boost his energy levels.

Lots of Water and Rest

Roughly 60 per cent of our body is made of water. Water maintains the body's fluid balance, helps transport nutrients, regulates body temperature and digests food. It also flushes out impurities and improves the skin, energy levels and brain function. John makes sure he drinks at least six glasses a day and rehydrates after a strenuous workout.

Sleep is just as vital to his strict regimen. John makes sure he sleeps for eight hours every day. Sleep helps repair the body. Muscles actually do not grow or tone during workouts. Rather, they grow afterwards, during peaceful and uninterrupted rest and sleep.

John's Daily Diet Plan

Throughout the day, John eats food that is low in GI (glycemic index). Due to his rigorous routine, he needs to nibble every two hours. He loves having salads, like lentil salads and quinoa salads, green vegetables, and seasonal fruits like apple, sweet lime, orange and musk melon.

His daily protein requirement is 200 g, after which he doesn't consume any more protein for the day.

Early Morning

John is an early riser. His day begins at 7 a.m.

He has four egg whites, one sweet potato and a seasonal fruit early in the morning and washes it all down with green tea.

After this he hits the gym for his routine workout. A rigorous session at the gym means he must have a sumptuous and balanced breakfast to regain his energy.

Breakfast

John has a breakfast, at around 9.30 a.m., of six or seven egg whites, slices of toast with butter, ten almonds and a glass of protein shake.

Lunch

He eats a balanced lunch, usually consisting of steamed fish, sprouts, vegetables, salad, yogurt and fruits like papaya.

Snack

He snacks in the afternoon on four or five egg whites, potatoes and citrus fruits like orange, grapefruit or sweet lime.

Dinner

John consumes small amounts of carbohydrates after sundown, because the body's metabolism rate slows down at night and there is every chance of carbs getting stored as fat.

John has a frugal dinner at around 9 p.m., which consists of a bowl of soup, rotis made from jowar (great millet) or bajra (pearl millet), fish and veggies.

He also takes multivitamins and supplements for essential oils and fats required to maintain a healthy balance.

Workout Routine

As a fitness freak, John hits the gym in the morning and works really hard to maintain his physique. His workout sessions—spread across six days of the week—focus on perfecting each part of the body. He takes Sundays off and simply relaxes on that day.

John's workout regimen—complemented by his high-protein diet to maintain his powerful, muscular body—is aimed at burning around 4000–5000 calories every day.

Monday

He begins his weekly workout session by exercising his chest and triceps. After a brief warm-up, he starts with 6 sets of bench presses. The bench press works the pectoralis major as well as supports the chest, arm and shoulder muscles such as anterior deltoids, serratus anterior, coracobrachialis, scapulae fixers, trapezius and the triceps.

Next, he does 3 sets of incline bench-presses and another 3 sets of decline bench-presses (15 reps each). Incline presses are effective for maintaining his big, bulky upper body, while the decline presses create the sharp lines. A combination of all three targets the muscles of the torso and gives a balanced appearance.

He follows this up with a short warm-up and then does free dumb-bell flyes to tone his upper-body muscles. These are strength-training exercises in which the hand and arm move through an arc while the elbow is kept at a constant angle. Flyes are done to work the muscles of the upper body. He follows this with 3 sets of cable flyes (15 reps), 2 sets of incline dumb-bell flyes and 2 sets of decline dumb-bell flyes (15 reps each).

He then changes his position to do 4 sets of triceps push-downs (15 reps) to strengthen the muscles in the back of the arm. He concludes the day's regimen with 3 sets of dips (15 reps). Narrow, shoulder-width dips primarily train the triceps, with emphasis on the anterior deltoid, the pectoralis muscles and the rhomboid muscles of the back.

Tuesday

John has earmarked Tuesdays for back and ab exercises. He begins with 4 sets of bent-over barbell rows (15 reps). This exercise is a great compound movement that incorporates the lats, rhomboids, rear deltoids, traps and the biceps. He then moves to 4 sets of pull-ups (15 reps), which strengthen the back muscles. The 4-set shrugs (15 reps) that follow target the trapezius muscles of the back.

Next, he performs 3 sets of leg raises and crunches (12 reps). Leg raises target the entire abdominal area, including the lower abs. Crunches, on the other hand, help tone and develop the side and front muscles of the torso, specifically the rectus abdominis and obliques. When performed regularly, this core-strengthening exercise helps improve balance, posture, athletic performance, and makes daily tasks easier.

Wednesday

John reserves this day for doing cardio exercises. Beginning with a treadmill sprint for half an hour, he goes out bicycling for twenty minutes.

He rounds it off with abdominal workouts for tightening his transversus abdominis, the deepest abdominal muscle, followed by lunges, which strengthen, sculpt and build several muscles, including the quadriceps (or thighs), the gluteus maximus (or the buttock) and the hamstrings. He finishes the day's routine with crunches.

Thursday

On Thursdays, John works on his legs. He begins with 4 sets of leg presses (12 reps). This exercise is specifically for the lower-body muscles. It works on the thigh muscles: the hamstrings in the rear and quadriceps in the front. The action of extending the hips works on the gluteus maximus muscles.

Next, he moves on to 4 sets of squats (20 reps). Squats exercise the entire body and help build lean muscle, and reduce fat.

John targets the lower back as well as the mid and upper back, specifically the erector spinae areas. He does 4 sets of extensions (15 reps) and 3 sets of leg curls, aka hamstring curls (15 reps). This is an isolation exercise that targets the hamstring muscles.

He ends the day's session with 3 sets of hack squats (15 reps). Hack squats, barbell or machine, are very conductive to hypertrophy.

Friday

John focuses on his shoulders and biceps on Fridays. He begins with 3 sets of overhead presses (15 reps).

This increases the strength of the shoulder region. He then does 3 sets of military presses (15 reps) to build and sustain a muscular, strong upper body, and push the shoulders to their limits.

John next moves on to 4 sets each of lateral dumb-bells and alternate dumb-bells (15 reps) to build his deltoids, the thick triangular muscle covering the shoulder joint, and used for raising the arm away from the body.

He then does 3 sets of hammers (15 reps). Hammers help sculpt the brachioradialis, biceps (brachii) and brachialis. The first is a forearm muscle, which sticks out when doing hammers. Biceps and brachialis are upper arm muscles. He rounds off the day's workout with 3 sets of standing barbell-presses (15 reps).

Saturday

On the weekend, John once again does cardio exercises. After 30 minutes on the treadmill, he bicycles for 20 minutes. He follows this up with exercises to tone his abdominal muscles and rounds it off with lunges and crunches.

Known as the pyramid workout, this is one of the most challenging exercise routines. The three basic exercises i.e., push-ups, lunges and crunches, work most of the muscles in the body.

On Sundays, John takes a break from his back-breaking routine and just relaxes.

Outdoor Activities and Martial Arts

John is an outdoor person and always tries to participate in games. He is very disciplined when it comes to workouts but keeps varying his exercises and changing his routine to avoid monotony. John has been following the rigorous regimen set by his personal trainer, Vinod Channa.

Channa is an extremely knowledgeable fitness expert, and John has been training with him since the days of *Force* in 2011. Channa devises new exercises for John to make the workout sessions interesting. Variation not only keeps things interesting but also keeps the body guessing as it adapts to new activities.

John tries to learn a new form of fitness every two to three months. He also wishes to train in Krav Maga, a self-defence system developed for the Israel Defence Forces (IDF) that consists of a wide combination of techniques sourced from judo, boxing and wrestling along with realistic fight training.

Three years ago, while shooting for *Rocky Handsome*, John trained in Silat, a martial art involving knives. John had to train for fourteen hours every day for two weeks. As a result, the action scenes in the film are amazing. They look professional, thanks to John's complete dedication in learning a new defence technique.

John has changed his body type for almost every single movie. Sometimes he is buff and sometimes lean—it is amazing to watch him transform. In order to make sure he does not face any health issues, John pays full attention to eating right and balancing his calorie intake. But he feels that no one should overdo it because that can have an adverse effect on the body. One should be aware of any body damage and take it easy in case of a sprain or strain or any other kind of injury. 'You should never work out when you have a fever or a viral attack. You will hinder both your ability to work out effectively and delay your recovery—a double negative,'[6] he says.

John has always believed that while it is nice to look good, one should strive to have a healthy mind and lead a responsible and honest life too. At the end of the day, six-pack and eight-pack cease to matter if one's outlook and attitude fail to live up to the physical perfection.

10

Sonu Sood: The Indian Arnold Schwarzenegger

Bollywood Background

Sonu Sood is one of the fittest actors in Bollywood at the moment and has a body that could give Arnold Schwarzenegger a run for his money. He's our desi Hulk. His trainer, Yogesh Bhateja, describes Sonu's body: 'Every muscle is more prominent and well-designed than ever before; his body today is even more shredded and ripped. In one word, he is well sculpted.' Visually, Sonu's body is very appealing. He is all biceps, six-pack and super-toned abs and not an ounce of flab.

In showbiz, one's body is as important as one's acting talent. Sonu is especially someone who has made his mark in the entertainment industry due to his spectacular physique.

Sonu has often said in interviews that being an 'outsider' and not a part of the Bollywood clans, he's had to work his way up and face many hardships. 'When you are an outsider, no one is ready to meet you or listen to you,' he says.[1] He was often dropped from films during his early years to make way for star kids. But thanks to his stunning physique, he's made a place for himself in this highly competitive industry. In 2010, he starred in the hugely successful film *Dabangg*, which had superstar Salman Khan playing the popular cop Chulbul Pandey, with Sonu as his antagonist, Chedi Singh. Sonu held his own against Salman and garnered loads of praise from critics and a huge fan following. At 6 feet 2.5 inches, and weighing 80 kg, he looks like the kind of man you wouldn't want to take *panga* with. From Moga in Punjab, Sonu is the archetypal *hatta katta* Punjabi *munda*. You can just picture him eating tandoori chicken and parathas with loads of butter, all washed down with tall glasses of creamy and frothy lassi. But his diet is far removed from the original Punjabi fare!

In 2013, he acted in *R . . . Rajkumar*, a masala action film directed by Prabhu Deva—renowned choreographer, film director, producer and actor—along with Shahid Kapoor and Sonakshi Sinha. The film was a big commercial success and saw Sonu Sood looking ripped and spectacularly toned. In fact there is even a line in the movie in which the protagonist Shahid Kapoor asks Sonu's character admiringly,

'*Bhaiya*, how much time did it take you to build a body like that?' Sonu himself is quite frank about his consistent hard work. It is something for which he has been working on for a very long time, since college, in fact. For him, gymming is a daily ritual, like eating food or drinking water. While studying engineering in Nagpur, he joined a gym and never looked back as far as his training was concerned. His childhood idols were Arnold Schwarzenegger and Sylvester Stallone, and he would dream of building a body like them one day. Over the years, Sonu has worked diligently to achieve his goals. He's also very up to date on fitness techniques and shares a very close bond with his trainer, Yogesh, who he feels guides him well and has been instrumental in shaping his body over the years since *Happy New Year*.

In 2014, Sonu was a part of this movie, which required him to look really muscular. The movie had an ensemble cast that included Bollywood biggies like Shah Rukh Khan, Deepika Padukone and Abhishek Bachchan.

In the movie, Sonu sports an impressive eight-pack that sometimes threatens to overshadow SRK's toned and whistle-worthy body! Sonu plays an ex-army guy who loves blowing things up. Armed with a dynamite body like that, he seemed quite suited for the role.

Happy New Year Workouts

Yogesh trained Sonu for *Happy New Year*, for which he was required to have a very ripped and muscular look. Sonu was extremely pleased with his efforts and the results are there for everyone to see in the movie.

He underwent rigorous training for the film, which required him to meticulously work on each part of the body, evident from the gruelling regimen outlined here.

These workouts are designed in such a way that the reps are decreased while the weights are increased. This form of training is known as hypertrophy.

Chest and Triceps

- Flat bench-presses: 14, 12, 10, 8, 6
- Decline presses: 14, 12, 12, 10
- Incline hammer-presses: 14, 12, 10, 10
- Pec decks: 18, 16, 14, 12
- Cable crossovers: 25, 25, 25, 25
- Trip cable pully push-downs: 18, 16, 14, 12
- Overheard tri ext with rope: 18, 16, 14, 12
- Skull crushers with dumb-bells: 18,16,14,12
- Reverse push-downs with cable: 18,16,14,12
- Hanging leg-raises: 25*6

- Russian twists: 50*4
- Planks: 1-minute alternate sides
- Planks: 1-minute, both sides, 3 times

Back and Biceps

- Lat pull-downs: 14, 12, 10, 8
- Body-weight chin-ups: 12*4
- Close pull-downs: 12, 10, 8, 6
- Seated rows: 12, 10, 8, 8
- Single-arm dumb-bell rows: 12, 10, 8, 8
- Underarm bent-over rows: 12, 10, 10,8
- T-bar rows: 12, 10, 8, 8
- Upper-back flyes: 18,16,14,12
- Pull-over with dumb-bells: 12, 10, 8, 8
- Hammer curls: 12, 10, 8
- Preachers: 12, 10, 8, 6
- Dumb-bell concentration curls: 12, 10, 10, 8
- Hyper ext: 15*4

Shoulders

Preparation exercises:
- Rotator cuff exercise internal and external, and overhead rotation of shoulders with resistance band: 15*4
- Rear-delt flyes: 14, 12, 10, 8

Supersets of these two exercises with dumb-bells one after the other:

- Overheard dumb-bell presses: 12, 10, 8, 6
- Front presses: 12, 10, 8, 6

Supersets of these exercises with dumb-bells one after the other:

- Side lateral-raises: 12, 10, 8
- Front raises: 12, 10, 8

Supersets of these exercises with cable pully one after the other:

- Face pulls: 12, 10, 8
- Upright rows: 12, 10, 8
- Shrugs: 12, 10, 8
- Full crunches: 200
- Oblique cable crunches: 150 each side
- Rotary torsos: 100 each side

Legs

- Free squats: 100
- Weighted squats: 14, 12, 10, 8, 6
- Leg presses: 12, 10, 8, 6
- Walking lunges with 20 kg dumb-bells: 24*4
- Dead-lifts: 14, 12, 10, 8
- Leg curls: 14, 12, 10, 8
- Leg exts: 12, 10, 10, 8

- Seated calf-raises: 12, 10, 8, 6
- Standing calf-raises: 18, 16, 14, 12, 10, 8
- Calf presses: 12, 10, 8, 6

He focused on two body parts in a day and worked out for six days in a week for *Happy New Year*.

He also concentrated on working out his abs almost daily.

Happy New Year Diet

Sonu has a lot of faith and trust in Yogesh as far as his training and diet recommendations are concerned. For this movie Yogesh chalked out a diet plan that would enhance his sculpted body without causing any unnecessary weight gain.

Sonu would start his day with either a glass of warm water with honey and lemon, or 30 ml of aloe vera in 300 ml of water/a big pot of water (water detoxification). Generally, Sonu does this water detox when he's not shooting; this is recommended when you don't have to go to work, and are generally at home as the body detoxes, as it may involve frequent trips to the bathroom.

After about thirty minutes, Sonu would eat 40 g of oats along with four boiled egg whites. After his morning workout, the actor would have a protein and apple shake.

The actor never worked out on an empty stomach as Yogesh felt that the intensity of the workouts required a certain amount of calorie intake to perform better. The egg whites gave him enough protein, and the oats provided the necessary carbs required for the energy he expended.

For lunch, he would have vegetable quinoa pulao or tofu salad with avocado, olives, kale, spinach, cherry tomatoes, cucumber, jalapeños, green peas, baby corn, asparagus and a spoonful of flaxseeds.

After three hours he would eat a vegetable omelette of five egg whites. Then, two hours later, he would have 50 g of fat-free Greek yoghurt with blueberries.

Dinner consisted of boiled or grilled vegetables like spinach, bell pepper, cucumber, broccoli, asparagus, baby corn, beans and carrots.

Just before going to bed, he would have a glass of casein protein shake. This helps build and repair muscle tissues when the body is at rest.

Sonu's Food Philosophy

Sonu is a vegetarian but not as hardcore as Shahid Kapoor. He does eat eggs, which work as a great source of protein. He also includes plenty of lentils and grains which round off his protein intake. He eats a lot of green vegetables, fruits and salad. Sonu is very health conscious and abstains from smoking and drinking.

His rarely indulges in cheat days because he feels that all the effort of working out so much shouldn't go to waste.

He feels it's important to eat at intervals and advisable to have six meals a day. This helps maintain a high metabolism. He prefers a light lunch of brown rice, dal and salad; although it keeps varying and can include oats and quinoa. For snacks, he prefers fruit salads and coconut water. He's given up his favourite meal of dal and rotis, as rotis add to water retention in the body.

If he has to look lean for a body shot or close-up shots, he avoids salt and carbs completely for a couple of days prior to the shoot. For *Dabangg*, he was on a complete salad diet.

Sonu also feels cutting down on carbs like rice and rotis helps him maintain lean muscle. Instead, he has oats. However, he does have brown rice in moderation.

It goes without saying that he avoids fried, oily and junk food. Sonu does have a sweet tooth though, so he cannot resist rasgullas once in a while. But he eats them only after squeezing out all the sugar syrup. This is his only weakness, for which he feels extremely guilty.

Undoubtedly, Sonu's sense of discipline and dedication is praiseworthy. It's a way of life for him and not just something he does before shooting for a movie or photo shoots. So let's have a closer and more detailed look at Sonu's normal or daily diet.

For breakfast, Sonu has half a cup of oats cooked with water and cinnamon along with one whole egg and two egg whites scrambled with spinach, bell peppers, onions, cooked in olive oil. This is accompanied by a glass of orange juice. The second meal of the day is a whey protein and almond milk smoothie, which he usually has post workout.

Lunch is usually a salad with tomatoes, bell peppers, avocados, spinach and 150 g of paneer/tofu. Sonu also has half a sweet potato along with the salad.

To make sure he keeps his metabolism high between lunch and dinner, he has an apple and a protein shake as a snack. The fifth meal of the day consists of 200 g of steamed broccoli with bell peppers, asparagus, baby corn, kale and 30 g of quinoa. Quinoa is high in protein and a great alternative to wheat. It has an excellent amino-acid profile and contains all the essential nine amino acids—including the elusive lysine and isoleucine acids—which other grains lack. It is also naturally high in dietary fibre, making it a slow-digesting carb and thus a low-GI option.

For his final meal of the day, Sonu has five boiled egg whites.

All meals are cooked in olive oil and not more than two to three teaspoons of oil are used throughout the day. Recently, Yogesh has introduced coconut oil to Sonu's meals. Coconut oil is high in lauric acid, a type of saturated fatty acid. Although this oil does raise cholesterol levels according to medical studies, it mainly increases HDL, the healthy cholesterol, in the body. This oil contains medium-chain fatty acids (MCFAs), which are used directly for energy by the body. It is also a source of essential fatty acids that helps the body absorb fat soluble vitamins such as A, D, E and K. Salt is used sparingly too, and black pepper, turmeric, green chillies and cinnamon are the only spices used to cook his food.

Yogesh confides that the only other occasion Sonu does cheat is when he visits his home town in Punjab. He indulges in rajma chawal or dal makhani and rotis. But this again is extremely rare. Yogesh is full of admiration for Sonu's determination and focus, and he feels that compared to other stars who do binge on a regular basis, Sonu is very committed to a healthy lifestyle.

As Sonu is completely into fitness and likes to keep up with the latest trends or research in training, he is always willing to try new things to enhance his fitness. To this end, Yogesh is going to put him on the ketogenic or keto diet. Yogesh explains, 'It's a high-fat, high-protein diet with minimal carbs. So it incorporates 45 per cent of fats, 35 per cent of proteins and 20 per cent of carbs only. It's much more healthy as it minimizes fat or doesn't allow the body to gain more fat because it utilizes the fats already present in the body.'

Yogesh is very optimistic about this diet and sees Sonu benefiting from it very much. The name keto comes from the body's increased capability to produce ketones in the liver to be used as energy. The reason behind this is that when you eat something high in carbs, your body produces glucose and insulin. Glucose is the easiest molecule for your body to convert and use as energy, so it is chosen over any other energy source. And insulin is used to process the glucose in your bloodstream by taking it around the body. Since the glucose is being used as a primary energy source, the fats in your body are not needed and end up being stored. So typically, on a normal high-carb diet, the body uses glucose as the main source of energy. By lowering the intake of carbs, the body is induced into a state known as ketosis. This is a natural process that the body initiates to survive when food intake is low. During this state your body produces ketones which are released from the breakdown of fats in the liver. The end goal of a properly maintained keto diet is to force your body into this metabolic state. This is not done through starvation of calories but instead through starvation of carbs. The human body adapts incredibly. When you overload it with fats and take away carbs, it starts to burn ketones as the primary energy source. Yogesh is a big proponent of this diet, and says, 'Optimal ketone levels in the body offer many health, weight-loss, physical and mental benefits as well as increased energy levels.'

Sonu's Fitness Approach

Sonu is very particular and focused about his workout routines. He rarely misses a day. He works out for six days a week and keeps changing his exercises every week. But the basic focus on body parts remains the same. Also, he prefers working with light weights and keeps increasing the number of sets instead of the weights.

When shooting in a place where a gym might not be available, he goes for long runs or walks. But he makes it a point to keep himself physically active every day. He also practises kick-boxing for fifteen to twenty days every couple of months.

Sonu knows there are no shortcuts to having a great body. It is only achieved by having a disciplined and consistent approach to your fitness and diet. He also feels it's very important to de-stress. He uses exercise as a great stress-buster to stay physically and mentally fit.

Let's take a look at Sonu's regular daily workout.

Sonu's Daily Workouts

(the number after the * reflects the number of sets for that exercise)

Day 1
Legs Workout
- Free squats: 25*4
- Overhead lunges: 24*4
- Leg presses: 12, 10, 8, 6
- Stiff-leg dead-lifts: 12, 12, 10, 10
- Leg ext: 14, 12, 10, 8
- Leg curls: 14, 12, 10, 10
- Standing calf-raises: 20*5
- Seated calf-raises: 12, 12, 10, 10, 8, 8
- Calf presses: 12, 10, 8, 8
- Pull-ups: 12*4
- Parallel-bar push-ups: 12*4

Day 2
Shoulders and Biceps
- Rear-delt flyes: 14, 12, 10, 8
- Overhead dumb-bell presses: 12, 10, 8
- Front presses with barbells: 12, 10, 8

- Side lateral-raise with cables: 14, 12, 12, 10
- Face pulls with cable/upright rows: 14, 12, 10, 10
- Front dumb-bell raises: 12*4
- Shrugs: 12, 10, 8, 8
- Alternate dumb-bell curls: 12, 10, 10, 8
- Preachers: 12, 10, 8, 8
- Hammers: 12,10, 8, 8
- Crunches alternately with 1-minute planks (multiple sets): 25*8

Day 3
Back and Triceps
- Seated rows: 14, 12, 10, 8
- Single-arm dumb-bell rows: 12, 10, 8, 8
- Close-grip pull-downs: 12, 10, 8, 8
- Wide lat pull-downs: 12, 10, 8, 8
- Bent-over row with barbells: 12, 10, 10, 8
- Upper-back flyes with dumb-bells: 14, 12, 10, 10
- Tri press-down/weighted diamond push-ups: 14, 12, 10, 8
- Tri cable pully push-downs: 12, 10, 8
- Overhead single-arm dumb-bell ext: 12, 10, 8
- Tricep kickbacks with dumb-bells: 12*3
- Hanging leg-raises: 25*6

Day 4
Chest and Calves
- Push-ups: 25*4
- Flat bench-presses: 12, 10, 8

- Incline dumb-bell presses: 12, 10, 8
- Hammer presses: 12, 10, 8
- Spiderman walks: 25*4
- Parallel-bar dips: 12*4
- Crossovers: 25*4
- Pec decks: 14, 12, 10, 8
- Weighted standing calf-raises: 18, 16, 14, 12, 10, 8
- Seated calf-raises: 12, 12, 10, 10
- Calf presses: 12, 10, 10, 8
- TRX knee-tucks: 50*4
- Russian twists: 50*4

Day 5
Free weights and Functional
- Push-ups variations (close, wide, elevated, archer, explosive, zigzag, single-hand)
- Pull-ups
- Parallel-bar dips
- Thrusters
- Explosive lunges
- Dead-lifts
- Battle-rope waves
- TRX knee-tucks and pikes
- TRX side-planks
- Spiderman walks

Day 5
Cardio and Stretching
- Walk: 20 minutes

- Sprints: 10 minutes
- Cross trainer: 20 minutes
- Cycle: 20 minutes
- Plank
- Shalabhasana
- Full-body active stretches

Day 6
Free Weights and Functional
- Push-up variations (close, wide, elevated, archer, explosive, zigzag, single-hand): 100 in total
- Pull-ups: 12*4
- Parallel-bar dips: 12*4
- Thrusters: 20*5
- Explosive lunges: 25*4
- Dead-lifts: 12, 10, 8, 6
- Battle-rope waves: 50*4
- TRX knee-tucks and pikes: 50*4
- TRX side-planks: 1-minute, each side, twice
- Criteria of choosing weights: Ensure that the last 2 reps of each set should be performed using one's best strength without support.

Apart from his daily workouts in the gym Sonu makes it a point to cycle 40 km every week. Yogesh says, 'He's very particular about cycling every week. Mostly he cycles to Siddhivinayak temple from his house in Andheri, Mumbai. When he's unable to do that, he cycles on the spinning cycle in the gym. But he's very particular about doing this once a week.' As far as focusing on muscles is concerned, Sonu and Yogesh either target hypertrophy or try to cut down on muscle mass, depending on the look required for a movie. The former involves working out to gain muscle mass. They use heavy weights with limited repetitions and one to two minutes of rest in between the sets.

In the second case, where the focus is to cut down on muscle mass and achieve a more shredded and ripped look, the training incorporates multiple number of reps like 18, 16, 14, 12. This focuses on multiple variations of the muscle, thus targeting each and every major or minor muscle fibre. Here multiple sets are performed and increased cardiovascular activity is included, like cycling, running, swimming, etc.

Sonu recently starred in *Kung Fu Yoga* which starred the extremely popular international celebrity Jackie Chan, and also Disha Patani and Amyra Dastur. As it is an action-packed film, as all Jackie Chan movies are, Sonu had a lot of action scenes in the movie. The director, Stanley Tong, said in an interview that, 'Sonu Sood has a fit body and is a fast learner when it comes to our action.'

For the film, Sonu went to Dubai to train in martial arts. Then during the shooting of the film in China, he was further trained by Jackie Chan's team of martial-arts experts. Along with this, Sonu continued his daily workout routine. He was required to gain muscle mass, which led him to do a lot of strength training and callisthenics.

His diet was mainly boiled vegetables like broccoli, spinach, kale etc. He also ate lots of soups, which contained many Chinese herbs. Sonu found himself adding black pepper in everything because it was extremely cold in China at the time of shooting. Also, black pepper helped keep the body's metabolism high. He snacked on dry fruits to keep himself warm. He would eat 35–40 g of mixed nuts every day that included hazelnuts, Brazil nuts and macadamia nuts.

To a large extent, Sonu followed his usual meal plan: eggs and quinoa and protein shakes. However, his calorie intake was increased through higher intake of proteins and carbs. Good sources of fats like avocado (80 g in a day), goat cheese and Greek yoghurt (50 g in a day) also were included.

Conclusion

Yogesh emphasizes that though it is possible today to have access to vast amounts of information regarding health and fitness, it is more important to be able to follow and maintain a routine. He also stresses on the inadvisability of trying to achieve a six-pack within a short period of time. It is very important to do this gradually rather than pushing your body to overachieve, which can then lead to injuries. Also it is very important to understand your body and its limitations and then work around them. So maintain a healthy and nutritious diet and follow a workout routine best suited to your body.

All in all, Sonu's commitment, dedication and passion for fitness is extremely inspirational. As he writes in one of his tweets, 'People who plan to go to the gym from next week or from Monday or from first of any month, are the ones who will never go. So, please go now before it's too late.' This is the message that one should take to heart; that fitness should be a way of life one should commit to as soon as possible.

11

Dev: God from the East

'The difference between the impossible and the possible lies in a man's determination,' announces the Facebook status of the man who embodies this statement, and he is none other than Deepak Adhikari, aka Dev. A multifaceted, multitasking genius, Dev is a film actor, producer, entertainer, singer, entrepreneur, restaurateur and, more recently, politician.

Born in Mahisha, a small village in Keshpur, West Bengal, in 1982, Dev did a series of odd jobs until he began his film career in Mumbai. He went from being an observer on the sets of Abbas–Mustan's thriller *Tarzan the Wonder Car*, to making his acting debut in *Agnishapath* in 2005. The film fell flat and so did Dev. But undeterred by failure and not one to give up so easily, he resurfaced the very next year with *I Love You* (2006), which met with lukewarm response from the public. The following year, he went back to Mumbai to sharpen his acting and other allied skills. He learnt to dance and trained under action choreographer Aejaz Ghulab. It was a turning point for him when he returned to Tollywood, he was a different man altogether, with an excellent physique and confidence oozing from every pore of his sculpted body. He never looked back again.

In 2008, Dev starred in three Bengali films—*Premer Kahini, Chirodini Tumi Je Amar* and *Mon Mane Na*—all of which went on to be megahits. Thus, a star was born. Since then, Dev has reigned over the hearts of millions of Bengali-film lovers. In 2009, he starred in four blockbusters: *Jackpot, Challenge, Paran Jai Jaliya Re* and *Dujone* and went on to become the proverbial Midas. It seemed as though every film that featured him would become a super-duper hit, grossing millions. However, not one to sit on his laurels, Dev turned his attention from commercial films to meaningful, art cinema. In 2010, he starred in Aveek Mukhopadhyay's *Ekti Tarar Khonje,* which was critically acclaimed. In 2013, he took up a challenging role in Kamaleshwar Mukherjee's *Chander Pahar* (Mountain of the Moon). Based on Bibhutibhushan Bandopadhyay's novel of the same name, the film traces the journey of young Shankar (Dev) from his rural village to Africa, in search of the fabled 'mountain of the moon', and its secret treasures of gold and diamonds.

Bringing Martial Arts to Tollywood

In 2011, *Paglu*, starring Dev and Koel Mallick, was released. Directed by Rajib Biswas, this movie was the biggest opener in Tollywood history before *Challenge 2* was released in October 2012. Dev introduced martial arts to Bengali cinema, something Tollywood had never witnessed before. The actor can be safely called the first martial-arts hero in the industry.

In an interview, the director of the film lauded Dev and said, 'Dev was superb with the action sequences. He did some martial-arts stunts and also learnt kick-boxing for two months only for my movie. I was amazed with his dedication. Bengali films never saw [sic] such action sequences before. There is a train and bike chase sequence that was shot by Zoyeb and Dev. I was literally scared when they were shooting this sequence without any body double. Hats off to their courage.'[1]

Dev's Regular Workout

Dev has a well-proportioned, muscular, athletic body only because his strict workout routine is tough and highly intense. Equally important for a physique like his is a nutritious diet. He has five to six small meals in a day to keep his metabolism rate going.

Dev starts his day at around 7.45 a.m., and the first thing he needs after waking up is a cup of piping hot tea served in bed. After this, he hits the gym and begins his workout routine with light warm-up exercises, followed by intensive physical training focusing on building muscle. Standing tall at 6 feet 1 inch, Dev's perfectly sculpted physique is every youngster's dream. Trained by celebrity fitness and nutrition expert Arnold Fudge, Dev follows his trainer's instructions to a T. Fudge has Dev do a combination of cardiovascular training along with body-weight exercises. This takes about two to three hours daily. Dev's body-weight exercises and workouts are mainly focused on his abs, arms and legs, and include cardio exercises, crunches, pull-ups, bicep curls, squats and leg lifts.

Dev starts the workout session with warm-up exercises. Fudge mixes and matches various exercises to keep monotony and boredom at bay. The warm-up session is followed by some cardiovascular exercises and heavy-weights training.

Fudge says, 'My workout pattern for my students varies from day to day, depending on his or her body changes and weak points. For example: I always follow the basics; if I realize my student's weak point is a chest muscle, maybe the lower pec, I always start with a decline press, parallel bar or flyes. Then I follow it up with flat bench-presses and incline bench-presses.' Fudge keeps doing this and working on the weak points, so that these become strengths.

For abs, Dev does bent-over barbell rows, pull-ups, shrugs, leg raises and crunches.

For his arms and legs, the movie star has to train with alternating dumb-bell lying triceps extension, kneeling push-ups, dumb-bell hammer curls, superman from floor, Russian twists and Swiss ball hip-raises and leg curls.

Dev also does pull-ups, push-ups, and crunches back to back, only resting between total sets. The day's workout regimen is finally wound up with dumb-bell dead-lifts.

For cardio, he is put on circuit-training workouts. These include in-between sessions of aerobic moves and strengthening muscle exercises, with minimal rest in between.

Fudge also employs high-intensity interval training (HIIT) for Dev, which involves drills like sprints, lunges and speed skaters with brief periods of rest in between. He also does polymetric exercises that include jump squats, burpees or box jumps. These are all methods of metabolic conditioning reliant on explosive movements and the goal is to contract the maximum number of muscle in the minimum amount of time.

After his workout is over, Dev has a tall glass of fruit juice as he relaxes with the day's newspapers and updates. This helps him regain energy and cool off.

Transformation for *Chander Pahar* and *Bunohaansh*

Dev has never hesitated to transform his body for a particular role. A very disciplined person, his strict fitness regimen and diet schedule is amazing.

Chander Pahar required Dev to totally change his look from a lanky village lad to a tough-as-nails, no-nonsense supervisor working with African and immigrant workers in the dense forests of Africa. Later, he again had to shed a lot of weight to project a famished, thirsty and critically ill Shankar, lost in the wilderness and on the brink of death. He reminded us then of Tom Hanks and his transformation for the movie *Cast Away*. To achieve that look, Dev cut down on carbs and depended on lean protein and protein drinks for energy. His hard work was paid off, and his acting skills were highly appreciated.

In 2014, Dev signed with director Aniruddha Roy Chowdhury to act in the thriller *Bunohaansh* (Wild Goose). Here too, Dev worked hard for his body transformation to suit the role of Amal, an honest, gullible, lower middle-class youth trying to make ends meet and falling prey to an international smuggling racket.

The same year, he took another daring decision when he chose to do *Joddha*. While filming, he had said: 'For the first time I am playing a warrior. In *Joddha,* my character, Rudrapratap, kills a hundred soldiers at a time! So, my body should be fighting fit.'[2]

Other than being fit, Dev worked hard every time to get into the skin of the character, whether for Amal in *Bunohaans,* Shankar in *Chander Pahar* or Rudrapratap in *Joddha*. 'Just having a dream body wasn't enough for my role as a warrior, I also had to pick up . . . the walk . . . the broad shoulders, broad chest, someone who walks with his head held high . . . at the same time, I had to get an attitude while talking.'[3] In *Joddha*, he had to capture the aura of a leader on the battlefield, out to lead his soldiers to victory. Thus, his body had to reflect that power of the heart and courage of the soul.

To achieve the warrior's body, Dev worked out in the gym, sometimes even at 2 a.m., every day, for four months. On certain days, he would begin at 4 a.m. However, he didn't follow a fixed schedule and worked out whenever he had time. He couldn't dedicate a fixed number of hours every day to exercise and bodybuilding, as he was simultaneously shooting for *Bunohaans* and *Bindaas*. Juggling his looks for the diverse roles was also a tremendous challenge.

Diet and Workout for *Joddha*

Despite being fit as a fiddle, Dev had to follow a special diet routine to get in shape for *Joddha* as he needed to put on muscle. To this end, he ate a lot of chicken and carbs.

Initially, his aim was to have a six-pack, but the director realized that for a warrior film set 400 years ago, a six-pack would not be relevant. Warriors in those days used to shield their bodies with iron jackets, instead of flaunting bare torsos. Hence Dev too had to cover the upper part of his body with a shield and the only time people got to see Rudrapratap's bare body was when he died.

Dev really enjoys his food. Dieting for him is a tough proposition. Hence, his trainer put him on a balanced diet.

For breakfast, he would have a protein shake, curd and fruits, which would be followed by a light lunch that included brown rice and chicken.

Dinner would consist of fruits and boiled veggies.

His gym regimen was equally tough, going through a plethora of exercises, including cardio, weight training and rigorous metabolic training.

The challenge was to return to his normal diet and exercise regimen post *Joddha* and control the craving for rice, mutton and sweets and retain the body he had worked so hard for.

How Dev Prepared for *Chaamp*

With *Chaamp*, Dev entered a new phase of his acting career. A blockbuster sports drama directed by Raj Chakraborty, Dev was the lead actor as well as the producer. Dev once again sought Arnold Fudge's help to transform his body. Fudge remembers the time when Dev called him. 'It was October 2016 when Dev called me up and I was then busy training and sculpting my own body to participate in the world bodybuilding championship. Hence, Dev had to wait for a while.' *Chaamp* also marked the debut of supermodel Rukmini Maitra as the female lead opposite Dev.

They started training from the end of January, and within forty-five days, Dev's weight went down from 100 kg to 80 kg, and he had muscle definition. This was all possible due to the actor's hard work and perseverance. With his busy schedule—as a member of Parliament and as one of the busiest actors of Tollywood—Dev made it a point to never miss his workouts. He was also careful about his protein and water intake. Fudge put him on a no-salt diet, which made sure that there was no water retention.

After witnessing his dedication, Fudge was completely impressed and moved by his perseverance. The trainer adds: 'I have never seen him do yoga, but yes [I had] definitely heard [about] him learn[ing] martial arts as a child. For his movie *Chaamp*, he learnt boxing and went for boxing classes to improve his punching skills and speed. I strongly believe that it is not the quantity of the workout but the quality of it that brings about results like his fit body in *Chaamp*.'

From his experience and expertise, Fudge believes there are several myths surrounding fitness. There are some who believe a rigorous workout in a gym is enough to be fit. He also mentions a rise in instances when overdoing exercises or overworking muscles have led to serious health issues involving ligament and tendon tears or even the cracking of bones. Similarly, crash-dieting is a complete no-no. According to Fudge, there are also unprofessional instructors who do not have proper training themselves nor are they certified to help train others.

Often Fudge comes across women and young girls who take to crash-dieting to lose weight. Fudge warns that the end result can be dangerous, especially for the body's immune system, which can be compromised if the body does not receive proper nutrition. Consuming just protein or protein shakes and salads and completely skipping carbohydrates is not a proper diet plan for those who live in a tropical climate. The typically excessive heat and sweat make it essential to include energy-giving ingredients in the diet plan. Thus, fitness is not a one-track race. Several factors together contribute to a fit body.

'My perception for achieving fitness and a good strong body is a proper blend of target workouts and diet to help my clients achieve their goals. For actors like Dev, the workout and diet regimen keep changing constantly as they have different requirements for different roles. For those who do not need such a change, I usually give them a target diet and exercise plan and keep adjusting it to keep it interesting.'

Dev's Diet

Fudge prescribes a balanced diet for Dev. He insists: 'We need to keep in mind that every body type is different and requires a different workout and diet regimen. Just by taking in protein and no carbs is wrong, as our body requires a certain amount of carbohydrates daily for energy and to function well. If excess protein is not used by working out, it will be converted to fat.'

This drives home the importance of training under someone who has the knowledge of balancing workouts and diet so that it doesn't harm the body. Also, what suits one person might not suit another. Therefore, one should never blindly copy diets and exercises; instead, it is recommended to have your own trainer help you do targeted exercises.

Dev follows a balanced diet set by Fudge. He abstains from junk and oily food. This helps keep his body toxin-free as much as possible and prevents fat accumulation. Fudge makes sure that whatever Dev eats is rich in proteins, vitamins and calcium. The diet chart is planned according to Dev's work schedule and his roles. When he is required to gain weight, he is allowed to have everything. Every day becomes his cheat day then. But on days he has to work out late at night after a busy shooting schedule, he has complex carbs to keep his energy levels high.

However, the main emphasis is on protein intake to maintain amino-acid levels, so that there is no muscle loss. Proteins are the best muscle-building ingredients of a balanced diet. Since Dev is often put on an intense workout regimen to build muscle tone, proteins automatically become essential for his body. But when he works out at night, like he did for *Chaamp*, he is directed to have almonds or a few slices of any seasonal fruit from time to time.

When Dev has to look lean in his films, he begins his day with oats and egg whites, and then hits the gym to do his cardio exercises, which are interspersed with an intake of protein shakes. Two hours after gym, when he goes out for shoots, he is given carbs and then at an interval of every two hours, 250 g of fish or chicken to make sure enough protein is consumed. This is followed by fruits or salads after another two hours. He prefers papaya, apple or pomegranate as these are lean, easily digestible and fortified with natural minerals like iron. As Fudge points out, there are instances when a client hogs on fruit salad, containing juicy fruits like mangoes and litchis, feeling like he is on a great diet. But fruits like mangoes are extremely fattening and, instead of doing good, can actually lead to the accumulation of body fat and an increase in weight.

Evening snacking and dinners are completely light for Dev. In the evening, he has vegetable soup since vegetables are a good source of fibre. Again, two hours later, he is served 250 g of fish or chicken to maintain the protein level at night. Fudge prefers that he has fish, since it can be easily digested and is fortified with omega-3 fatty acids, which are considered to be the best antioxidants by doctors.

Fudge outlines that the basic strategy for any diet plan should be dividing meals into six or seven portions a day. If Dev feels hungry before hitting the bed at night, he has a bowl of sour curd to kill his hunger pangs.

But it is not just his body, but also a heart of gold and a life of discipline that sets this reigning actor of Tollywood apart. Dev has reached the pinnacle of success only through dedicated hard work and a disciplined approach to everything he does. His life is an inspiration for all those who think dreams are not attainable. Dev's humble beginnings and his phenomenal rise to superstardom show that if one dreams big and puts in all effort to succeed, they will hold the world in their fist one day.

Dev is currently riding high on his success after his second home production, *Cockpit*, created a massive impact at the box office, and he is now breaking all records with Bengal's costliest film, *Amazon Obhijaan*. Dev is all set to release his home-production film *Kabir* this year. Needless to say, he is the top hero of the Bengali film industry with a fan following of millions.

Notes

Chapter 1: Hrithik Roshan: A Lean, Mean Fighting Machine

1. Anuradha Chaudhary, 'Fitness Alert—How I Got My Body Back In Shape', *Times of India*, 14 September 2014.
2. Ibid.

Chapter 2: Challenging All Fitness Limits: The Aamir Khan Way

1. Kriti Saraswat, 'Aamir Khan's trainer reveals how he got the *Dhoom 3* gymnast's body!', The Health Site, 8 September 2014.
2. '*Dhoom 3* My Toughest Role So Far: Aamir', IndiaTimes.com, 1 November 2013.

Chapter 4: Varun: Dhawan and Only

1. Sharanya Manola, 'Behind the Hot Body of Varun Dhawan Lie These 6 Unique Fitness Secrets and

His Strict Diet Regime', BollywoodShaadis.com, 8
February 2018.

2. 'Varun Dhawan's Workout Routine and Diet: Fitness
    Tips Straight from His Trainer', NDTVFood, 16 May
    2017.

3. Archana Iyer, 'This is How Varun Dhawan Prepared
    for His Role in *ABCD2*', *Health & Nutrition*, 28 July
    2015, http://bit.ly/2FUHmTW.

4. 'Varun Dhawan's Workout Routine and Diet: Fitness
    Tips Straight from His Trainer', NDTVFood, 16 May
    2017.

5. Archana Iyer, 'This is How Varun Dhawan Prepared
    for His Role in *ABCD2*', *Health & Nutrition*, 28 July
    2015, http://bit.ly/2FUHmTW.

6. 'Varun Dhawan's Body, Workout Routine and Diet',
    IndianBodybuilding.co.in, http://bit.ly/2FULhjF.

7. Ibid.

Chapter 6: Tiger Shroff: The Sculpted Dancer

1. 'Hrithik Roshan Praises Tiger Shroff for his "Michael
    Jackson" dance', India TV, 8 September 2014.

Chapter 7: Bipasha Basu: Abs-olutely Gorgeous

1. 'Bips, the Lady Goonda!', *Times of India*, 30 August
    2009.

2. Bipasha Basu's Facebook page.

3. Maike Steuer, 'I am Obelix minus the belly: Bipasha
    Basu', *Mumbai Mirror*, 6 January 2013

4. Ibid.

5. Id.

6. 'Arthritis in early age is a battle: Bips', HealthyDunia. com, 3 September 2013.
7. Maike Steuer, 'I am Obelix minus the belly: Bipasha Basu', *Mumbai Mirror*, 6 January 2013.
8. 'My mantra is to work out for heart and soul: Bipasha', *Indian Express*, 6 February 2010.
9. A superset is when one set of an exercise is performed directly after a set of a different exercise without any rest in between.
10. Priyanka Parab, 'Bipasha Basu: From Flab to Abs!', MediManage.com.
11. Ibid.

Chapter 8: Shahid Kapoor: Fiery and Fit

1. Interview with Abbas Ali, Shahid's trainer.
2. 'Shahid Kapoor, Varun Dhawan grateful to Shiamak Davar', *Times of India*, 10 April 2015.
3. Interview with Abbas Ali.
4. Ibid.
5. Id.

Chapter 9: John Abraham: Body of Work

1. Swagata Yadavar, 'Want a body like John Abraham? Here are his tips', MediManage.com, http://bit. ly/2G5adIv.
2. Ibid.
3. Id.
4. Somya Abrol, 'John Abraham tells us how he keeps his skin healthy and glowing', IndiaToday.com, 9 August 2017, http://bit.ly/2FTyAWd.

5. 'Fitness Tips', JohnAbraham.com, https://bit.
   ly/2H5GmOl.
6. Shikha Shah, 'Fitness is my only drug: John
   Abraham', *Times of India*, 4 January 2014, https://
   bit.ly/2Efbh7J.

Chapter 10: Sonu Sood: The Indian Arnold Schwarzenegger

1. In conversation with Sonu Sood.

Chapter 11: Dev: God from the East

1. 'It's Too Cold to Shoot in Paris Now: Dev', *Times of
   India*, 11 January 2017.
2. Kushali Nag, 'Mr Muscles', *Telegraph*, 13 September
   2014.
3. Ibid.